Naturally Healthy Woman

SHONDA PARKER

Loyal Publishing
www.loyalpublishing.com

Naturally Healthy Woman

Loyal Publishing, Inc.
P.O. Box 1892, Sisters, OR 97759

Copyright 2001 by Shonda Parker

WARNING-DISCLAIMER

Cover art by Robert Duncan, Robert Duncan Studios

ISBN: 1-929125-28-3

This book is dedicated to my daughters,
Emily, Eryn and Eliana

May you always rejoice in the way you were created:
Woman.

Contents

ACKNOWLEDGEMENTS

As always, this book is really the work of the many people who have taught me along the way, who have shared their stories and personal healthcare journeys with me, and the experts who shared their vast knowledge, so that I might pass along some of it to you.

I especially thank the friends who happily responded to my many calls asking, "Does this sound okay? Will this really help women?": Jackie Peacock, Wendy Wilkins, Lolo Long, Vivian Mock, Nicole Alders, Shelley Treadway, Susie Roberts, and Rebecca Berry. They are all very dear to me, and I hope still willing to receive my calls.

My pastor, Steve Wilkins, has been a greater help than he will ever know. I thank God for Pastor Steve's faithful preaching of the Word, which has solidified much of my belief about health and the responsibility of stewardship.

Much of my learning regarding women's healthcare is due to these professionals: Micki Cabiniss, M.D., David VanderMolen, M.D., Lynn Marie Myers, M.D., Donna Kolar, M.D., Donna Miller, CPM, Ann Crowell, CPM, Susan Hulet, CPM, Margie Spence, CPM, Al Faigin, D.O., Nancy Park, R.N., Becky Law, R.N., I.B.C.L.C., Susan Whisman, CPM, Fred Cummings, M.D., and many others whom I have encountered over the years in various teaching settings. Credit for the factual information in this book goes to them, for their teaching, and for guiding me to good resources. Any errors are mine alone.

On both a personal and professional level, I am particularly indebted to Dr. Micki Cabiniss, M.D. of Western Carolina Maternal Fetal Medicine Clinic in Asheville, North Carolina. Dr. Cabiniss taught me the areas of evaluation used in investigating the causes of recurrent miscarriages (Part Three, Chapter 3), when she evaluated my husband Keith and me after our ninth miscarriage. I am grateful for her willingness to see me and evaluate me when I could get no other physician to delve into our history of pregnancy loss. She ministered to me in a profound way during a very difficult time in our lives, and walked me through an education that allows me to share her wisdom with you in this book. Dr. Cabiniss is the type of physician all physicians should aspire to become.

Lou Anne Jensen invited me to speak in 1989 to a group of women in Tarrant County, Texas, at what later became a nonprofit organization, Informed WomanCare, dedicated to educating women about their choices in childbirth. This book began with that speaking engagement, my first on this topic. I thank Lou Anne for all the years of her friendship, love and encouragement. This book is the culmination of what we started those years ago.

My dear friend, Tana Basinger, has provided me with an enormous amount of encouragement over the months of writing. I hit a lull when I should have been busy with research and writing, and Tana managed to cheer me out of it by continually telling me the book was needed "right now!" and that I was the one to write it. I thank her for being such a devoted friend.

My family has been wonderful, particularly during my final week of work on the manuscript. The children were kind enough to take on my chores, and my beloved husband, Keith, has been diligent in cooking our meals or bringing food home, rubbing my aching back, massaging my toes, and doing so many other wonderful things for me. I love them all, and thank God for the gifts they are to me.

INTRODUCTION: BLESSINGS OF HEALTH

The beauty of womanhood is a glorious thing to experience. When we are able to rejoice in our design and calling as women, the fullness of our days becomes manageable. This only happens as we understand and appreciate the way we are made. The Naturally Healthy Woman was written to help us know our bodies better: how the female body functions and what measures are open to us when it is not functioning normally. It is not only about natural health, or conventional health care. It is about womanhood—about what is unique and beautiful in our design, and how we can learn to be stewards of that design.

I have been interested in health since I was a young girl, because of its importance to my mother. She taught me all she knew about maintaining health. By her assertive example, in doctors' offices and hospitals, she taught me about the need to understand the process of healthcare, and the need to keep pushing for answers when something is not right. This was a great gift.

Health is active. Informed WomanCare is a way of saying: "I am willing to take responsibility for my health, to be a good steward of my body, to be a partner in my healthcare with my professional healthcare provider, rather than letting things happen to me as a silent participant."

I hope to give each of my young daughters the vital gift of knowing how to be a steward of the wondrous creation that is her body. This is just as important for me, and for you. I should not give way to whatever my flesh wants, and then look for someone to heal me. Natural health tells me that what I do every day both to, and for, my body, is an important part of my health.

Sometimes, conventional medical care offers little other than life-disrupting drugs and surgery. When conventional medical care is necessary, the ideas in this book will help women make that into a more positive experience. However, natural medicine can offer a variety of means that do not disrupt life, but instead, increase vitality. Read, study, learn, look at yourself honestly, and become an informed, Naturally Healthy Woman.

Shonda

THE LADDER APPROACH TO HEALTH^{TM}

The Ladder Approach to Health will already be familiar to those who have read my previous books. This concept is based on the idea that health is maintained by following the health practices outlined in God's holy Word, the Bible, and that we repair our health through a step-by-step process. As we climb the ladder of repair upward from the least interventive means, our risk increases. There is little risk of injury if we fall off the first rung; if we fall off the top rung, our risk of injury is great. This increase in risk may become necessary in some situations, in order to repair areas of heavy damage, or in acute health crises.

Top rung: Surgical Intervention

"Big-Gun" (High Toxicity) Pharmaceuticals

Low Toxicity Pharmaceuticals

Botanical (Herbal) Medicine

Physical Medicine/Nutritional Changes

This ladder approach acknowledges the aspect of rebuilding in attaining health. Having climbed the ladder to repair problem areas, we generally will need to use the therapies on the lower rungs as we descend. Restoration to health often involves using a combination of therapies. The sooner we begin to intervene when an illness begins, the less intervention we probably will need to use.

Many times we can solve our health concerns with a simple change in diet or lifestyle (physical medicine). The next step up involves using herbs for healing—botanical medicine. We do not have to be fearful of herbs as medicine, but we do need to respect their chemical components, and become knowledgeable about their medicinal actions.

Some health crises may require us to climb the ladder above botanical medicine into pharmaceuticals. Again, we do not have to fear pharmaceuticals to the extent of never using them for medicine. We can read about the effect a particular pharmaceutical has on the body, seek professional counsel and make an informed decision, weighing risk against benefit. The key factor in home healthcare is knowing when to seek professional help.

Obviously, we must obtain pharmaceuticals or undergo surgery under the guidance and care of a licensed physician. Often, those who begin to practice nutritional and botanical medicine eschew any form of allopathic medicine, including any use of pharmaceuticals. I believe this to be unwise. Our acknowledgement of the great benefits of allopathic medicine in crisis situations is an important aspect of relaxed and confident family healthcare. The comfort of knowing I have alternatives, if my home care is not succeeding, or if I have encountered an illness so acute that home measures would not have time to work, allows me to practice with greater confidence. Nutritional and botanical medicine are not alternative forms of medicine. They are essential and foremost forms of medicine. Allopathic medicine is the alternative that we can be thankful is available when necessary.

Sources for products recommended throughout *The Naturally Healthy Woman* are found in the Resource Directory at the end of Part Seven. Shonda does not receive any remuneration for recommending or promoting sales of any of these products.

HEALTHY FOUNDATIONS

What is health?

Health is not contained in a drug, a pill, an herbal medicine or a hormonal cream. Health is total, involving body, mind and spirit. A healthy woman wakes up in the morning looking forward to another day of serving God, praying to gird herself for the day's work, and listening to God's voice in His Word. She is a good steward of her body, taking care to eat nutritious foods and recommended supplements. She laughs at her children's delightful escapades, shares her thoughts with a friend, snuggles next to her husband while reading at night, and revels in her relations with him before contentedly closing her eyes for a restful night's sleep. Health is much more in the heart than in the broken toe.

Our attitude forms the foundation for our health. The city slogan of Asheville, North Carolina, is: Altitude with Attitude. An attitude to health might instead be: Attitude with Altitude. We should set our minds on things above, not on earthly things. Yet, how can we do this when our bodies are undeniably earthly things until the day of Jesus Christ?

My body His Temple

If I believe that I am in control of my own destiny, my spirit is burdened when I have a health problem. This in turn produces more health problems. If I believe that God will not let me get sick if I eat all the right things, take all the right supplements, and pray in the right way, and then I get cancer, either I have to blame someone or something else, or I have to question my whole belief about God. If, on the other hand, I believe my sole purpose is to glorify God, that my body is His temple, to feed both spiritually and physically until that day when sickness and death will be finally conquered, just as our Lord Jesus Christ has already conquered spiritual death, then I will live each day seeking the glory of my Lord, not merely my own health and comfort. I recognize that there is no health within me. Health must always come from the Father through His Son. Only when we understand that can we greet even cancer with an attitude of health.

We cannot create health, any more than we can do any good thing apart from the grace of God. When we eat grains, and natural meats, fruits and vegetables, we are not creating health; we are obeying God's command to be stewards of His creation. He can choose to bless us with a body free from disease, or choose to allow disease for the sake of His glory, as He did with Job and the apostle Paul. It is a glorious, amazing glimpse of grace to see someone who has endured personal loss, disease, or a life of hardship, continue to see her Lord as the "giver of all good things." Everything that comes to us, the Lord says in His Word, is good for us. Everything. Knowing this allows my "attitude with altitude" to prevail. My health, like my faith, is not dependent upon my circumstances, but completely dependent upon the will of my Father, who has a plan for my good that brings Him glory—a plan that has been in effect since the foundation of the world.

Once we have our spiritual foundation firmly fixed, we can proceed to the issues involved in the stewardship of His creation—our bodies. This stewardship is accomplished through healthful food choices, bodily exercise, and the regular, mysterious feasting on the Body of the Lord Jesus Christ through the communion meal, or Lord's Supper.

Choose the whole foods diet

Research continues to confirm that the best choice we can make regarding our food intake is to eat plentiful grains, fruits and vegetables. This does not mean we must completely avoid meat, but meat should not be the main portion on our plates. As naturally healthy women, we will look on a porterhouse steak, with a baked potato dripping in butter, as a once-in-a-great-while indulgence. We know that a high-fat diet increases our risk of heart disease, cancer, osteoporosis, and a host of minor ailments.

Eating whole foods refers to eating foods as close to their natural state as possible. This is not because we worship the natural state. The natural state of things is fallen. But research shows us that the more refined food products we eat, the higher our risk of menstrual complaints, as well as all forms of cancers. On the other hand, there are foods that will cut our risk of disease. In particular, certain foods can reduce our risk of developing breast cancer, a disease that statistics say will hit one out of ten women. The list below is comprised of foods that contain cancer-fighting substances, and that increase immune health, gastrointestinal health and bone density. They also help to decrease the mental "fog" that heavy foods tend to produce, and supply nutrients for maximum energy levels.

Twenty foods that reduce cancer risk and improve general health:

1. Carrot juice: carrots are packed with nutrients, but the cell walls must be broken down in order to release them. That means chewing until you drop on carrot sticks! Carrot juice is a better choice. An 8-ounce glass—with no additives or sweeteners, and the fresher the better—supplies 700% of our daily beta-carotene requirement. Baby food is another good source (yes, really). The process of pureeing the carrots for toothless infants makes the beta-carotene super-absorbable.
2. Daikon radishes: this type contains indole-3 carbinol, which lowers levels of a type of estrogen that may promote breast cancer.

3. 1% milk (preferably not the kind containing hormones and growth stimulants): milk fat contains conjugated linoleic acid, which fights breast cancer, both in test-tube studies and in mammals.

4. Tomato juice: supplies lycopene, a compound that lowers rates of breast cancer.

5. Broccosprouts: contain high levels of SGS, a compound that fights breast cancer tumors in mice.

6. Grape juice: has more cancer-fighting antioxidants than any other juice.

7. Salmon, tuna and anchovies: are rich in omega-3 fats. Women with higher tissue levels of omega-3 fats have a lower incidence of breast cancer.

8. Cherries: contain perillyl alcohol, a compound that may inhibit breast cancer in mice.

9. Orange juice: contains limonoids in the peel and white membranes, which inhibit breast cancer cells in test-tube trials.

10. Whole grains: studies show that women who eat refined grains have a higher incidence of breast cancer. The difference could be due to the daily consumption of bran from whole grains, which helps lower breast cancer-promoting estrogen.

11. Butter is better: choose small amounts of butter (which also contains milk fat) instead of trans-fat margarines, which increase the risk of breast cancer.

12. Green tea: contains antioxidants, and is rich in GCG, a compound that inhibits breast cancer cells in mice.

13. Olive oil: apart from its great taste, has been shown to lower the rate of breast cancer in women who indulge in it.

14. Garlic: kills breast cancer cells in test tube studies. Let it rest 10-15 minutes before heating. Heating right away doesn't allow time for the cancer-fighting compounds to develop.

15. Spinach: in one study, women who ate a serving of spinach at least twice weekly had half the rate of breast cancer of the women not eating it.

16. Veggie burgers and sausages: should replace much of the red meat in a healthy woman's diet. Red meat, particularly very well done, forms compounds that increase cancer rates among big meat-eaters.

17. Flaxseed: has 75 times more lignan precursors, compounds that inhibit breast cancer tumors in animals, than any other food.

18. Nuts and seeds: contain essential fatty acids that help lower breast cancer rates.

19. A daily multivitamin/mineral supplement, with vitamin D: a lower incidence of breast cancer is observed in women who take vitamin D.

20. Pure water in abundance daily: water increases the rate at which waste moves through the bowel, which in turn reduces the amount of toxins reabsorbed into the bloodstream. It also reduces the time those toxins come into contact with the intestinal wall, which reduces the risk of colon and breast cancer.

Whole foods for whole health

This list gives an idea of what "whole food" eating is about: substituting whole foods for processed ingredients.

WHOLE FOOD	IMITATION/PROCESSED VERSION
freshly ground, wholegrain flour	packaged white, wheat, rye, barley, or oat flour
purified water	sodas like Coke, Dr. Pepper; etc.
unsweetened fruit juices: fresh squeezed is best; then frozen; bottled is least desirable	juice "cocktails" or "drinks;" powdered, artificially-flavored drinks like Kool-Aid
herbal teas (no caffeine); green tea (caffeine)	black tea (caffeine); coffee
whole wheat pasta, spelt pasta, sesame pasta, etc.	white pasta
brown rice; buckwheat; millet; barley; rye; oats etc.	white rice; other refined grains
whole grains: whole, freshly cracked or rolled	boxed cereals; processed grains
wholegrain toasted bread crumbs	boxed croutons
wholegrain crackers	white flour crackers
unrefined oils: cold-pressed, extra virgin olive oil	hydrogenated fats and shortenings; refined oils
butter	margarines; spreads
goat milk; tofu milk; certified raw milk	homogenized, pasteurized milk

WHOLE FOOD	IMITATION/PROCESSED VERSION
certified raw milk (naturally white) cheese	dyed, added-to, homogenized, pasteurized cheeses
plain, live-cultured yogurt	sweetened or frozen yogurt
cultured dairy products	uncultured, sweet dairy products
unfiltered, unpasteurized apple cider vinegar	distilled vinegar
baking powder without aluminum or yeast	baking powder containing aluminum
low sodium baking powder (aluminum-free)	baking soda
carob powder	cocoa; chocolate
uncooked, unfiltered raw honey: ½ cup = 1 c sugar; Grade A pure maple syrup; unsulfured molasses; fruit juices/purees; dried raw cane juice; fructose in small amounts	white sugars: sucrose, dextrose, glucose, and "raw" sugar; corn syrup; brown sugar
baked chips; popcorn; dried unsulfured fruits; raw nuts; granola	fried chips; sulfured dried fruits; candy; snack items with added sugars, dyes, preservatives, or other additives
organic fruits, vegetables and grains	conventionally-grown fruits, vegetables and grains
unhydrogenated peanut butter, made with 100% peanuts without added sugar (or salt, if preferred); sesame butter (tahini); cashew butter; almond butter	commercial peanut butter and other nut butters
raw, lightly steamed, or grilled vegetables	boiled or fried vegetables
raw fruits	canned or frozen fruits with added sugars
clean animals (according to Leviticus 11) that can be completely bled: the common ones we eat are chicken, turkey, deer, and beef (in moderation)	animals raised on chemically-treated grains and hay, and fed chemicals to keep them (supposedly) "healthy"
beans, peas, lentils, whole grains, etc.: the majority of protein should come from vegetable sources	meat, particularly red meat

This list is not intended as a hammer upon your head! It gives you an idea of the type of foods—whole foods—that make up the largest portion of a Naturally Healthy Woman's diet. Indulgences on the right side of the chart are quite acceptable, every once in a while, in a healthy person's diet.

> ***Remember: It is not what you eat every once in a while that will cause your health problems. It is what you eat every day.***

The Naturally Healthy Life

Life is so much more than simply the foods we eat. We are not machines that merely need the right oil or fuel to function properly. We are made up of body, mind, and spirit. A large part of our health is a direct result of our spiritual health. As we discussed at the beginning of this chapter, how we view our world and our God is vital. If we worship God in fullness and with reverence, that attitude will be reflected in full and abundant lives that are glorifying to God.

As women, our lives are often full of an overwhelming number of daily tasks. They can wear down our desire to worship, and our ability to do so with a clean heart. All busy-ness, with no time for physical and spiritual refreshment, makes for a dull woman! We need to address some areas of practical home, and time, management.

Housework is NOT just women's work

The home environment, caring for husband and children, is a woman's domain. However, it is a faulty idea that every job in the house belongs to the woman. In our family, my husband rightfully fulfills his biblical place as head of the home. He has ultimate authority regarding the "doings" of our household and family. We call him our CEO. I rightfully fulfill my place as "chief operations officer" for the home, taking responsibility for everyday management. Our children are all vital "senior staff" with responsibilities of their own. I oversee them day to day, and seek out the advice and intervention of our CEO when necessary. I provide him with daily reports of home operations. We hire consultants and independent contractors as necessary, to look after jobs we are unable to attend to ourselves. Our home structure keeps the biblical structure of authority in place, while allowing those under authority the freedom to perform their duties in ways that best suit their own abilities.

The Family Corporation

The practical working out of our home structure is that all of us know our duty, and our responsibility to complete that duty daily. Anyone in business knows that the busiest person in a corporation is the Chief Executive Officer. Greater responsibility makes for more work. CEOs rarely spend all their working time in their own corporation's offices; they must travel extensively to oversee the corporation's financial health, product growth, and market stability. In our family "corporation", the CEO may travel every day outside the home to ensure his family's security. Although he is a busy man, he still has to pick up his dirty underwear from the floor, and is responsible for clearing up the trail of clothes he leaves behind him when he changes on returning to the home front in the evening.

The best leaders are those who know how to roll up their sleeves and fall in with the line workers to boost morale and get a big job done. Home CEOs know that they must do the same. There are times of big to-dos around the home that require a willingness to roll up the sleeves and immerse the hands and arms in a dishpan or toilet bowl. These incidences do not take away from his honor. Rather, they knit a special bond between family members as they work together to prepare for weekend guests, or to put on that big barbeque party.

Another challenge our CEO may face is effectively managing those times when his spouse is physically unable to carry on with all of her regular responsibilities, even though she may still be able to oversee family operations, her primary duty. He can evaluate the children to see if they are capable and ready to take on more responsibility, or he may decide to hire outside help, for a limited time period or indefinitely.

This may be a hard decision, as husband and wife discuss whether to do what they can on their own, or to take on the financial burden of hiring outside help. The essential element in this decision-making process is the recognition that the family has the moral freedom to hire as much outside help as necessary. There are many instances related in God's Word of godly families that had both male and female servants to help with running their households. As long as financial resources can be diverted from other areas to cover the expense, this is a totally acceptable way of doing family business.

Time Out

One of the biggest challenges that a CEO faces is learning how to love and value those for whom he is responsible. Although we all want our corporation's employees to have a good solid work ethic, the best of leaders know how to inspire people, not only through working with them, but also by giving them opportunities for the sheer enjoyment of living. Providing regular days off from the usual routine is essential. What better day for this than the Lord's Day? Every week we have the opportunity to spend a day resting in worship of our Creator and Lord, as well as time for family fun, in whatever manner the family members enjoy most. This may be a round of golf for some; for others, it may mean having a party. The principle is the same: take some time out to enjoy life. Even our Lord Jesus took time out, and urged His disciples to do the same.

The value of daily work to health

A woman's list of tasks is a long one. Every day there are yesterday's clothes (or more) to wash, meals to prepare, dishes to wash, a home to clean of clutter, dust and dirt, home management calls to make and receive, perhaps even business dealings to accomplish. If God has blessed the family union with children, they must be cared for and nurtured emotionally and spiritually, and educated, at home or in a private Christian school, so that their education is biblically founded. Every day there are the same tasks, the same responsibilities. And it is not enough for us simply to do them. We are commanded, in whatever we do to do it heartily, as unto the Lord (Colossians 3:23). That means with gusto, and without complaint! Now, how do we find the energy to do so much, with gusto, and think we cannot ever complain? It is not always easy to be consistent in living out that daily obedience. But it is possible.

Going forth with grace

We start with solid spiritual feeding each day: Bible reading, prayer, and meditation on God's Word. We tackle our duties with the awareness that we depend fully on God's abundant grace to help us accomplish them. That does not mean that we wait until we "feel" God's grace on us before we begin performing those tasks. Never! We get on with the job. As we go forth in obedience, we can trust in God's grace for the fulfillment of those duties in just the way He has planned for us. Trusting in Him brings peace, rather than anxiety about the number of things we are trying to accomplish. As long as we are diligent, He will bring about all that He desires for us, each day. This certainty gives comfort and energy in and of itself.

There are times of physical limitation for all women. In my latter pregnancies, there have been times when I have needed outside help to keep things running smoothly in the home. This has inspired me to work harder in between pregnancies to train my children in the daily operations of the household, so that now they can accomplish quite a bit without outside help. The point is this: whatever my physical abilities are, I need to have a "going forth" task list each day, to help me get started on those things for which I am responsible. Whether I have a cleaning lady, a cook or a nanny, I still need to see that the house gets cleaned, that meals are cooked and the children are cared for according to our family's requirements.

The value of friendship to health

Another area of spiritual feeding that we all need is our covenant community, the community that is formed of our brothers and sisters in Christ. We need others, and they need us. God's Word speaks of the value of friends. God our Savior, Jesus Christ, calls Himself a friend to us. Neglecting the importance of having someone whom we can call if we are in need is dangerous to our spiritual and bodily health. This covenant community means more than having a "best friend." It is made up of many people, far and near, who are joined with us in life in Christ. While they may differ from us in some areas of thought, and in their traditions, as long as they agree with us in the essentials of our faith, their worth is inestimable.

If we really think of our brothers and sisters in Christ, our close friends, as invaluable, then we will not allow small matters to grow until they drive a wedge between us. When we share in the covenant of Christ, we are sharing a relationship that goes beyond hurt feelings or casual friendships. We may live in a world made up of disposable items, but godly friends are not disposable. Our spiritual, and therefore our physical, health, is damaged if we walk through life making and dropping friends on the basis of matters outside of the essential doctrines of faith.

Spiritual health, spiritual healing

The Bible teaches us that we do not have a right to be angry with a bother or sister without cause, but we are to be reconciled with anyone who has something against us before we can cleanly come before the Lord (Matthew 5:22-24). We are also taught that there are steps we must go through when someone has sinned against us: first, we go to that person alone, to try to win him back; then, if he refuses to hear us alone, we take witnesses; then, if he refuses to listen to them, we are to bring him before the church. Finally, if he refuses to listen to the church, he is to be considered a heathen, not a brother (Matthew 18:15-17). There are many such verses regarding the need to control our anger, to put aside the self-love that makes us want to esteem ourselves more than we esteem others, and the need to forgive those who have offended us and ask for forgiveness. We should see one thing most clearly: whether we have sinned against a Christian brother or sister, or they have sinned against us, we have the responsibility to go to them for reconciliation and restoration. We do not have the option of waiting for time to heal our wounds. Time does not heal untreated wounds; it allows them to become infected, and the infection to spread throughout the body. Such an infection can destroy the physical body. In the spiritual realm, it is as true for the Body of Christ.

Restoration in the church means bringing a repentant brother or sister back into fellowship as fully as though there had never been a problem. Our fellowship may even be better than what we enjoyed before. If a friend has sinned against us, confessed, and repented, and we have forgiven her, we have the responsibility to restore her to our fellowship. We do not have the option of deciding to forgive, and then carrying on without restoring the friendship. That is not forgiveness, nor is it covenantal living. Restoration may not be easy, but it is better than the bitterness that, without it, is bound to grow within us. As to the health effects of bitterness, the Bible is quite clear: A merry heart doeth good like a medicine: but a broken spirit drieth the bones (Proverbs 17:22). Nothing breaks the spirit like the bitterness of a broken friendship.

The value of regular worship

One of the most vital contributions to our health is the corporate weekly worship with our brothers and sisters in Christ. We are commanded not to forsake the assembling of ourselves together (Hebrews 10:25). This verse refers not merely to having Christian friends and doing things with them: we are to assemble together frequently in corporate worship, so that we may exhort and encourage one another to hold fast to the faith and to be good works (Hebrews 10). This regular assembling together to worship our Lord binds us together visibly in our covenant with Him. We quickly recognize that our lives are not individual: we are part of a Body. What I do affects you, and what you do affects me. This limits our freedom to behave in ways that are unbecoming to Christ. We do not sin in isolation. My sin infects the entire Body of Christ. How wonderful to be part of such a Body, where we are kept accountable for our actions, and where our joy in the Lord is shared abundantly.

The feast before us

It is during this weekly worship that we eat the meal that affects our health most tremendously: the communion meal, or the Lord's supper. This is not a meal only in remembrance of Christ's sacrifice for us, and His cleansing of us as He brings us to Him. This is the meal in which we mysteriously feed upon the body of Christ and the blood of Christ. Even though we are not literally eating Christ's flesh and drinking His blood, we are in some mysterious communion with the Savior as He feeds us, His children. It is a means of grace for us, a feeding that fortifies us to go forth with our commission to further His kingdom. When we share regularly in this meal, we show in a tangible way our covenant with Him, and with those in His body. It shows to whom we belong. This meal also reminds us of the One who gives us our health. Since we have no health within us naturally, we see in this meal Him who feeds us, who creates and maintains our health. What a beautiful feast to look forward to each week.

Part One:
Divine Design

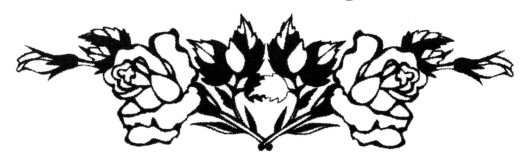

CHAPTER 1
PRE-PUBERTY HEALTH CARE

The health of our daughters, and of our daughters' daughters, begins in the womb.

Wait a minute! Isn't that a heavy responsibility to be placing on us when we may not be feeling well enough to eat healthfully? Yes. But it is a fact. All the internal organs of a female child, including ovaries and eggs, are formed in the first trimester of pregnancy. At the time of birth, a baby girl's ovaries contain almost 500,000 potential single-cell eggs, which will begin to ripen at menstruation.[1] If God blesses her with children, they will come from those eggs. Since almost everything an expectant mother takes into her body, through eating, breathing, or through her skin, reaches her baby through the placenta, every choice she makes during pregnancy will affect, not only her daughter in the womb, but her daughter's daughters as well.

HEALTHFUL PRENATAL CHOICES

Planning to give our daughters a healthful heritage begins when we make good health choices prior to pregnancy. A woman cannot know the time when God will choose to open her womb. A married woman of childbearing age should begin immediately to develop dietary and lifestyle habits that would be good for a baby, should God bless her in this special way.

Make certain the diet is made up primarily of whole foods nutrition:

We discussed the concept of whole foods nutrition in Healthy Foundations. What it means is that we try to eat foods that are not highly refined or processed. Whole foods nutrition is made up primarily of a plant-based diet; however, there is nothing wrong with eating meat, unless certain health conditions make eating animal products unwise. If the majority of a woman's diet consists of animal foods, this increases her risk of developing cancer, and increases stress on major body organs. We should also be concerned about low-dose antibiotic or hormonal residue in meats. We can try to make the best choices from these conventionally-raised meat offerings, or, if the budget allows, choose to buy naturally-raised meats. Some meat brands advertise that they contain "no fatty chicken," or that they were "not raised with antibiotics or hormones." These may be the brands we choose over others in the grocery store.

The biggest challenge for most of us is in becoming diligent about getting our minimum of five fruits and vegetables daily. Over the lifetime of a woman, overcoming this challenge is worth it for the health benefits, which include: weight control, a reduction in the risk of developing all cancers, heart disease, and osteoporosis, a feeling of well being or health due to nutrient intake, good overall body system health, and increased immune response. What could be a more excellent starting place for pregnancy?

Have a Toxic Metal Screen:

Environmental toxins known to be associated with the development of birth defects are: toxic metals, methyl mercury, lead, cadmium, organochemicals, DDT, dioxin, Agent Orange, and polychlorinated biphenyls (PCBs). Anyone who lives in a city, or who lives or works in an industrial environment, should be screened for toxic metals. This screening may be done through blood tests or a hair mineral analysis. Blood tests are more reliable for what is currently circulating in the blood, while hair analysis gives a better picture of low levels or of toxic metal buildup in the system. Your best choice in having these tests is to go to a nutrition-oriented care provider, one who is trained to evaluate the tests and make recommendations based on the results.

Switch to non-toxic household cleaners:

Frankly, I am a disinfectant nut. I like knowing I've got the biggest "gun" possible for wiping out the nasty, microscopic bugs that lurk in our kitchens and bathrooms. But I do resolve, when I know pregnancy is possible, and certainly during pregnancy, to stay away from those cleaners. I usually purchase a citrus disinfectant that is pretty powerful itself, and use milder cleaners in areas that don't need heavy disinfecting. These types of cleaners may be found in your local health food store, but often on supermarket or wholesale warehouse clubs shelves as well.

Avoid unnecessary drugs:

All nonessential drugs and medications should be eliminated, with the advice and assistance of a healthcare provider. Those that are essential should be evaluated as to the risks versus benefits for mother and baby.

Evaluate contraception use: Some contraceptives can be harmful to a conceived baby, either affecting normal development, or terminating life in the womb:

1. There is research to indicate that contraceptive foams, gels and suppositories may damage healthy sperm, although not enough to make it impossible for the damaged sperm to penetrate the woman's released egg and fertilize it.
2. The intrauterine device (IUD) has definitely been shown to be an abortifacient: this means it does not stop conception, but works by preventing the conceived baby from implanting securely in the wall of the uterus.
3. Many women, and even their physicians, are surprised to learn that the birth control pill can act as an abortifacient as well. It is supposed to act in preventing ovulation, but this action is not perfect. Many of us know women who have become pregnant while taking the pill. A fertilized egg equals a conceived baby.
4. The pill also works by preventing the normal monthly buildup of the uterine lining, where a baby would implant. If a pregnancy occurs, it may abort, as the baby is not able to burrow into what should be the thick wall of the uterus.

These contraceptive concerns need to be considered during the childbearing years.

Limit Caffeine Intake:

So far, studies on caffeine seem inconclusive in terms of its effect in lowering fertility, and in contributing to miscarriage. However, the effect of caffeine on the body is undisputed: it is a stimulant affecting metabolism, adrenal function, circulatory ability and the nervous system. Caffeine stimulates the adrenal glands to produce more adrenalin, constricts blood vessels, causes the shakes from nervous system stimulation, and speeds up the metabolism. Caffeine is a main ingredient in many weight-loss diet plans because of these effects. This alone should warn us against ingesting too much caffeine when preparing for pregnancy, because pregnancy is definitely not the time to be speeding metabolism to lose weight.

Caffeine occurs naturally in black tea, green tea (Camellia sinensis), coffee beans, cocoa (chocolate), cola or kola nut (Cola nitida), guarana (Paullinia cupana, which has two and a half times more caffeine than coffee), and mate (Ilex paraguariensis). Of course, it is also found in some soft drinks. The pharmacological effect of caffeine can be experienced from 50 mg upward; in doses exceeding 250 mg, these are likely to be significant. A study published in the American Journal of Obstetrics and Gynecology in January 1985 reported that women who consumed more than 150 mg of caffeine per day experienced an increase in spontaneous abortions (miscarriages). One 5-ounce cup of coffee can provide 150 mg of caffeine, depending on how it is brewed. Caffeine also has an antagonistic effect on important vitamins and minerals, lowering or preventing the absorption of nutrients, such as iron and zinc, from our food. Both of these are extremely important for fertility and childbearing.

When reducing or eliminating your caffeine intake, wean yourself slowly, over a period of weeks. This will decrease the withdrawal symptoms of headaches, fatigue and nausea.

Engage in a lifelong "Smoke Out":

Smoking depletes the body's supply of vitamins and minerals. It is also a constant irritant to the respiratory passages, and has been implicated in numerous diseases. Smoking during pregnancy may lead to miscarriage, prematurity, or intrauterine growth retardation, which causes low birth-weight babies. Although some women subscribe to the "I smoked during all my pregnancies, and none of that happened before" philosophy, these women and babies are the exception, not the rule. I realize that those who smoke are addicted to the drug effects of the cigarettes, and that it is difficult to overcome the addiction. However, I believe that any addiction, to nicotine, caffeine, drugs or food, can be overcome with prayer, determination, and the conviction to do what is best for you and your baby. If your husband smokes, he should quit too, for his own sake, and also because secondhand smoke is detrimental to mother and baby.

Limit or eliminate alcohol intake:

Even moderate alcohol consumption during pregnancy has been identified as the causative factor in fetal alcohol syndrome (FAS). This syndrome is characterized by growth retardation, and mid-facial hypoplasia: general flattening, short nose, and upturned, small eyes. There may also be microcephaly, mental disorder, and abnormal palmar creases. The toxicity may be caused by the alcohol itself, or by the breakdown products, such as acetaldehyde. The risk of fetal alcohol syndrome should discourage fertile women from consuming too much alcohol.

A woman who finds herself pregnant and knows she has had some alcoholic drinks since the conception does not need to spend the next nine months in despair. Many factors beyond our control may damage a baby's health. The key is to avoid those that we can control. Don't drink if you are planning for pregnancy, or if you know you are pregnant. Once again, hopeful fathers should also avoid alcohol during the preconception time period, as alcohol may affect sperm health.

Address current health concerns:

Any health problem or concern a woman has during her childbearing years should not be ignored, or she may end up having to endure that problem during pregnancy, making for more discomfort, and possible health problems for her baby. It is more beneficial to do a good laboratory analysis prior to pregnancy, with follow-up prenatal lab work during pregnancy. This allows a woman time to make necessary changes in her diet to ensure a healthy conception and early organ development time for her baby. It also alerts caregivers to health problems that need to be treated. Screening for toxoplasmosis, in addition to regular labs, may be beneficial to those who own cats.

Take supplements for maximum preconception care:

1. Begin taking a quality prenatal vitamin and mineral supplement, with absorbable forms of the nutrients. It should have at least 400-800 mcg of folic acid, 30-50 mg of iron, and 20-35 mg of zinc.
2. A supplement supplying essential fatty acids is important for correct baby development. Good sources are flaxseed oil, Evening Primrose oil, or blackcurrant oil.
3. An herbal source of minerals is an excellent choice to supply the macronutrients necessary for the functioning of the glandular system: it should contain nutritive herbs such as alfalfa, kelp, spirulina, and red raspberry.
4. If morning sickness was a problem during a previous pregnancy, milk thistle extract (standardized to contain at least 70% silymarin) is of great benefit to aid in liver function. Recommended amount: 3 per day.
5. An herbal whole-body cleanse is a good way to prepare for pregnancy, and beneficial to anyone with toxic metal content, sluggish bowels, liver or gallbladder problems. A good cleanse will last from 2 weeks to 1 month, and will not keep you on the toilet constantly. Any cleanse performs best when combined with a whole foods diet. An herbal cleanse should be done at least once a month prior to conception.

Further pregnancy preparation and care may be found in my book The Naturally Healthy Pregnancy.

HEALTHY CHILD CARE

Breast is Best:

Breast milk supplies all the necessary nutrients for a healthy baby. It is quite rare for a woman to be unable to provide adequate breast milk for her child. If, for any reason, breastfeeding problems are encountered, a Certified Lactation Consultant should be called. She will know best how to help a new mother establish a good milk supply.

Breastfeeding helps a woman to lose weight after her baby's birth, gives her baby the healthiest food possible, reduces food and airborne-induced allergies, reduces the risk of serious intestinal and respiratory infections during infancy, and, as an added bonus, does not produce the smelly bowel movements of formula-fed babies. The act of nursing increases bonding between a mother and her infant, and may also increase the child's intelligence quotient.

Food introduction:

Once a baby's teeth are coming in, it is good to have a plan for food introduction, like this simple plan which has worked for all five of our children: root vegetables first—carrots, sweet potatoes, beets, etc.; then fruits, such as apples, pears, plums, and bananas. Once the baby is a year old, we progress to whole grains. Meat and dairy products are not introduced until the molars come in, around 18-24 months. Our family philosophy is: if the baby does not have teeth to chew it, she does not need to be eating it.

Whole foods and essential supplements for girls:

The same food recommendations for mothers and fathers apply to young girls as well. They need a diet rich in whole foods, and low in refined and processed food products. If family meals come mostly from boxes, cans or frozen platters, that needs to change. Over a period of weeks, start adding fresh fruit, vegetables, and nutritious homemade meals to the household diet. This does put extra demands on a woman who may already be overwhelmed by all she has to do in a day, but it is possible to learn how to provide healthy meals to our family, without losing our minds, and our own physical well being, in the process. A detailed plan, and an explanation of Naturally Healthy™ eating, may be found in my book, Naturally Healthy Living: Real Food for Real Families, co-authored with Vickilynn Haycraft, the Whole Foods Digest "Mama."

I consider a daily multivitamin and mineral supplement essential for a young girl's health. Choose one that does not contain calcium, as this is best given as a separate, liquid calcium/ magnesium supplement each evening. The more a girl's bones are calcified prior to the onset of menses, the greater the reduction in her risk of developing osteoporosis later in life. If she gets an adequate amount of calcium through diet and supplements, she will not only want to, but also be able to, "rise up, and call us blessed" when she is seventy and her bones are still strong and solid.

CHAPTER 2
THE ONSET OF MENSES

GOD MADE WOMAN . . .

The first menstrual cycle can be an exciting time for a young girl, if we, as parents, help her understand the beauty of how God has created her, and how she is growing into womanhood. The normal onset of puberty occurs between the ages of 10 and 16.5 years, so we have several years of body changes that precede menarche (the onset of menstruation) to prepare our daughters for their first period.

One to four years before menarche, there is a sharp rise in pituitary hormone in the body, as well as increasing amounts of estrogenic and androgenic hormones. These internal changes correspond to secondary sex changes such as breast development and the growth of pubic hair.[1]

A growth spurt occurs prior to menarche that causes a young girl's protein requirements to be three times that of an adult. This growth will continue after menarche, but will proceed much more slowly, adding only, at most, two more inches to a young woman's stature. This means that girls who begin menstruating at an early age are likely be shorter than their later-blooming peers.[2]

When a young woman reaches menarche, those 500,000 eggs she has carried around since birth assume an active role. Each one of those cells that ripens into an egg is nourished by nearly 5000 others that will never ripen. Every month, one hundred to one hundred and fifty eggs will begin to ripen, with only one reaching maturity, capable of being fertilized. From the time of her first period until the cessation of menses at menopause, a woman may carry up to 4,000 ripe eggs.[3] What an absolutely amazing process!

The Hormonal Cycle

Normal menstrual cycles have two phases: a follicular (ovary) or proliferative (endometrium) phase, beginning with the first day of menstrual flow and culminating in ovulation, and a luteal or secretory phase, which ends with the onset of menstruation, the discharge of blood and the disintegrating endometrium. This function depends primarily on three endocrine sources: the hypothalamus, the anterior pituitary gland, and the theca granulosa cells of the ovary.

The Follicular Phase

A neurochemical transmitter, known as gonadotropin-releasing hormone (GnRH), is produced in the hypothalamus, and then carried through the portal vessels to the anterior lobe of the pituitary gland. This action results in the production and release of the gonadotropins FSH (follicle-stimulating hormone) and LH (leutinizing hormone) from the anterior pituitary cells. These hormones are transmitted to the ovary, where they stimulate follicle development and ovulation. The production of FSH and LH by anterior pituitary cells is not steady: there is a continuous secretion of pulsating discharges of the hormones, governed by cyclic changes in ovarian estrogen and progesterone secretion.

Estrogen (estradiol [E_2]) is the principal modulator of hypothalamic-pituitary activity. In the first few days of the menstrual cycle, estrogen levels are low. This stimulates secretion of GnRH, which in turn causes the release of FSH and LH. These hormones stimulate the follicle to begin maturing to become a ripened egg. Estrogen levels increase to aid the egg ripening process, and continue to increase until they peak just before ovulation. The increased estrogen levels work to inhibit FSH secretion, and the sharp estrogen peak acts on the hypothalamic-pituitary system, stimulating LH, and, to a lesser extent, FSH, release. Estrogen triggers the mid-cycle surge of LH, which induces ovulation.

The Luteal Phase

LH continues at a lower level of production after ovulation, helping to support the growth of the corpus luteum. Secretion of progesterone (P_4) increases rapidly after ovulation, with a concurrent, but lesser, increase in estrogen production. High levels of progesterone are maintained until about day twenty-three or twenty-four of the cycle, when the corpus luteum begins to regress if the egg (ovum) has not been fertilized. Since ovulation occurs mid-cycle, about day fourteen in a normal twenty-eight day cycle, and the egg has only twenty-four hours in which to be fertilized after release, corpus luteum regression corresponds to the time when the body recognizes that a conceived baby (fertilized egg) has not been implanted into the prepared uterine lining (endometrium).

As the levels of estrogen and progesterone drop, following corpus luteum regression, the endometrium that has built up in preparation for a baby begins to disintegrate. Menstruation follows. The low levels of estrogen and progesterone once again allow another cycle to begin.

By His divine design

When we understand our divine design, we can be grateful to our Creator for this marvelous process, rather than railing against the monthly hormonal changes that are designed to nourish and protect our unborn children, even before they are conceived. As Psalm 139 tells us, we truly are fearfully and wonderfully made. Before this process begins for our daughters, we can discuss with them how our bodies function, how we are divinely designed, and what we can expect during our monthly cycles. They need to know from us what this technical hormonal production and action process actually means for them, in practical terms, every month.

The menstrual cycle starts with the beginning of blood flow. This may be light initially, changing to a heavier flow during the next couple of days. Some women experience a heavy flow at the onset of menstruation, which lightens considerably during the next few days. Average menstrual flow is five days, with a normal range of from three to seven days. The flow is usually dark red, with some particles of disintegrated endometrium.

Normal menstrual flow has a characteristic musty odor. Good hygiene is important to cut down on odors. This does not mean using douches, feminine sprays or powders: it simply means daily bathing or showering. Douching after menstruation is also unnecessary: the vagina produces its own natural cleansing discharge.

No mysteries

Being prepared for menstruation is important to young girls. Talk with your prepubescent daughter about using sanitary pads or tampons. If her first period starts when you are not around, she will be comfortable getting what she needs. It is a good idea to see that she carries a pad in her purse at all times. Even once her regular cycles are established, she should be prepared for what will always be an unknown time of flow.

Menstruation has never been a mystery in our home. My daughters have seen what occurs, and brought boxes of sanitary pads to me when necessary. We have discussed it regularly, not in special "talks," but as a part of everyday living. They know what to expect when their own time of menarche arrives.

Sanitary pads are probably better than tampons, or a menstrual cup, for a young woman at menarche, when her vaginal opening is not much larger than when she was a baby. She also needs to get used to what her body is doing before venturing into the brave new territory of inserting any item vaginally.

Twelve is the average age for the onset of menses. A physician's opinion should be sought if menstruation begins before age ten, or is delayed until after the sixteenth year.

CHAPTER 3
CYCLE REGULATION

A SOLID FOUNDATION

Women experience cycles that range from twenty-one days to forty-five or as long as sixty days. Some have cycles that do not follow any regular pattern at all. This may not be much more than an inconvenience to a woman who wonders when her new cycle, with blood flow, will begin. However, irregular cycles can be indicative of health problems, hormonal imbalances, or may be a factor in infertility.

If you have irregular cycles that are suspected as a cause of infertility, your best step is to begin diagnostic laboratory work with a gynecologist or reproductive endocrinologist. They can do blood hormone tests and, if necessary, endometrial biopsies, to help rule out serious health problems. If all tests come back normal, or indicate only a slight hormonal imbalance, we can then try a natural therapy course before proceeding to more interventive means.

The foundation to menstrual health, in my opinion, is found in cycle regulation. Regulating cycles is not as simple as taking nutritional supplements or crèmes; rather, it is a whole approach to the way we live our lives. For instance, many scientific studies affirming the efficacy and safety of hormone replacement therapy (HRT), when using estrogen only, are questioned when they fail to account for the fact that many of the women in the study have a healthier lifestyle than the average woman. This may partly explain their better health. A solid health foundation will send a message to many symptoms to "pack up their bags and leave." Other symptoms may need months of work, and involve a commitment to changing nutrition, dietary supplements, and lifestyle habits.

With this foundation in mind, what can we do to bring about regulation in our menstrual cycles? One of the primary causes of cycle irregularity is a hormonal imbalance between estrogen and progesterone. Many things can contribute to this imbalance, but what often occurs is an excess of estrogen over progesterone. This excess is broken down in the liver, but, when the liver cannot process all of it, we end up with some fairly unpleasant symptoms. This is not to say that the liver is the key to hormonal health, but it is an important part of it. As we saw in the last chapter, pituitary balance is also important, given the pituitary gland's vital role in the production of female hormones.

LADDER APPROACH™ TO MENSTRUAL HEALTH

Our foundational level for relieving menstrual cycle problems begins with dietary and lifestyle intervention.

Dietary intervention:

- Limit the amount of animal foods, particularly during the cycle's luteal phase, from ovulation to the onset of menstruation. This recommendation arises from research showing that a vegetarian diet has been observed to prevent or lessen PMS symptoms (Abraham, 1987). Compared with those who eat meat, vegetarians excrete two to three times more estrogen in their feces, and have 50% lower mean plasma levels of unconjugated estrogens (Goldin, 1982). Broccoli, cauliflower and cabbage, members of the Brassica genus, contain a chemical that promotes the inactivation of estrogen (Michnovicz). Animal products, by contrast, are sources of arachidonic acid, a precursor to PGF_2, which inhibits progesterone synthesis (Abraham, 1984).
- Add complex carbohydrates, such as whole grains, legumes and lentils.
- Include deep-sea fish several times a week, for their essential fatty acid content.
- Add natural fats, such as avocados, nuts and seeds, but do not take in more than 15-20% of calories from fat.
- Eat a green, leafy salad each day.
- Choose fruits and vegetable of all colors: e.g. carrots (orange), broccoli (green), eggplant (purple), squash (yellow), cauliflower (white).
- Avoid caffeine, which can cause anxiety, irritability and insomnia.
- Avoid refined sugar, which causes hypoglycemic-like symptoms that complicate menstrual irregularities.
- Adhere to a whole foods diet. This is an absolute must. A whole foods diet is naturally high in fiber, which increases estrogen binding and excretion. Since the estrogen to progesterone ratio is typically elevated in menstrual problems, increasing dietary fiber to eliminate excess estrogen is theoretically helpful.

Nutritional supplements

The following are only the foundational basics for cycle regulation. This should not be taken as a comprehensive guide to nutritional support of the various menstrual concerns.

Basic multiple supplements: A basic multiple must include the following vital nutrients:
1. Vitamin A: 10,000 IU daily in a half-and-half ratio of vitamin A to beta-carotene if pregnancy is a possibility. When there is no possibility of pregnancy, up to 25,000 IU or more may be taken daily during the luteal phase of the cycle
2. B-complex: 50-100 mg daily of the various B vitamins
3. Manganese: 3-5 mg daily
4. Magnesium: 400-500 mg daily
5. Calcium: 1,000 mg daily
6. Vitamin E: 300-600 IU daily
7. Omega-6 fatty acids: Evening Primrose oil, 1.5 g twice daily
8. Vitamin C and flavonoids: 500-1,000 mg daily
9. Iron: 30 mg daily

Good choices for basic multiple supplements: Women's Forte by NF Formulas (also called Prenatal Forte); Opti-Gyn by Eclectic Institute; Woman's Choice by Enzymatic Therapy.

Vitex agnus-castus (Chaste berry): One of the finest and most beneficial herbs for women's reproductive health, vitex is used for: general reproductive health, PMS, heavy or frequent menstrual cycles, amenorrhea, certain types of infertility, lactation and menopause. Vitex seems to resolve PMS symptoms, irregular cycles, and heavy or frequent menstruation, by increasing progesterone levels and decreasing prolactin levels. This also helps in cases of infertility relating to hormonal imbalance. Even though vitex lowers excess prolactin levels, it is beneficial in increasing the flow of milk in breastfeeding women. I think vitex is a must for women with any type of menstrual cycle imbalance.
1. To establish regular menstrual cycles, a standardized product is recommended, at a dosage of 1-2 capsules, taken at approximately the same time each morning, or a standardized extract, at 40 drops each morning. Typical standardization for vitex is to 0.6% agnuside.
2. For crude herb capsules or tablets, 650 mg may be taken up to 3 times daily.
3. For a tincture: 40 drops may be used up to 3 times a day.
4. Chaste berry tea may be drunk: 1 cup 2-3 times a day.

Interaction Alert! Do not combine vitex with dopamine-receptor antagonists.

Liver support: An efficiently functioning liver is essential to hormonal health. The liver is responsible for detoxifying the body from excess amounts of hormones in the system. In a foundational program for cycle regulation, it is helpful to add a liver-supportive herb, such as dandelion or milk thistle. For mild liver stimulation, dandelion is a wonderful choice. For liver support and protection, milk thistle, standardized to at least 70% silymarin, is my choice. Either of these herbs may be taken with each meal during the day.

What if I get pregnant while I am taking dandelion or milk thistle? Dandelion has no known contraindications for pregnancy or lactation. However, it should not be used by persons having obstruction of the bile ducts, gall bladder empyema, or ileus. If you have gallstones, you should use dandelion only after consulting with your physician. On rare occasions, contact allergies caused by sesquiterpene lactones in the latex have been observed.

Milk thistle is considered safe for use during pregnancy, and has a long history of use by nursing mothers. People with diabetes who are taking milk thistle should monitor their blood glucose levels carefully, as they may need to reduce standard anti-hyperglycemic drugs.

Exercise: A regular exercise routine is beneficial for all of us, but a reasonable amount of exercise may be particularly helpful in dealing with menstrual irregularities. Too much exercise can induce amenorrhea, and too little exercise may allow excess amounts of estrogen to remain within the body, producing a plethora of menstrual woes. Walking is an exercise almost all of us can manage, if we are ambulatory. I try to take a break from household duties several times a day to walk around the neighborhood at a brisk pace. These are not long walks, but they provide me with several aerobic exercise opportunities daily. As a result, I have lost several pounds, an additional health benefit, and have the particular enjoyment of chatting with friends I run into during my walks.

A WHOLE LIFE PROSPECT

Achieving regular menstrual cycles means taking a look at your whole life for needed changes. Women who approach those changes one week at a time usually manage better than those who try abruptly to change everything in their life, only to become discouraged over the cheesecake missing from their diet. After changes have been soundly implemented, it is fine to enjoy times of splurging. Once cycle regulation has been achieved, some of those "splurging" foods may be enjoyed on a more regular basis, provided that the problem symptoms do not return.

Part Two:
Well WomanCare

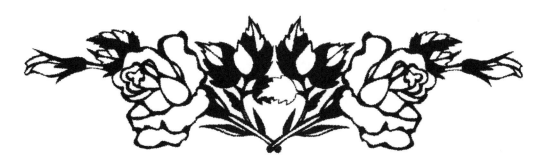

CHAPTER 1
WELL WOMANCARE

One of the areas we neglect the most as women is our Well WomanCare: careful health monitoring all the time, not only when something is obviously wrong. We may make ourselves visit the obstetrician/gynecologist's office once every year or two for a pap smear but, other than that, we simply leave well enough alone. This attitude can be dangerous to a woman's health. On the other hand, informed personal care may save her life.

Consider the woman who goes to her gynecologist or midwife, has her biannual pap smear, but never checks up on the test results. She goes on with her everyday life until debilitating vaginal bleeding and pelvic pain cause her to revisit her physician. Physical examination of the cervix reveals carcinoma—cancer of the cervix—that has already progressed beyond the cervix into the lymphatic channels, lowering her possibility of a total cure.

Or consider the woman who never does monthly breast exams. This woman does not even want to look at her naked body in the mirror, let alone examine each nook and cranny while palpating every inch of her breasts and underarms. The thought of a yearly checkup by a gynecologist or midwife increases her stress, so she neglects to go for four or five years. And then, the mere idea of having her breasts smashed and irradiated during a mammogram keeps her from having that examination as well. She is happily going about her life until, one day as she dries off after her shower, she cannot avoid noticing a large, immovable lump in her breast, with dimpling on her breast. When she does finally decide to have the lump checked out, she is told that she is in for a big battle for her life.

A Naturally Healthy Attitude

These two women are more the norm than the exception. Contrast them with our Naturally Healthy Woman. She observes her body each time she gets out of the bath or shower. She knows where her moles are and what they look like. She does her breast exams every month, at the same time during her cycle, so that she is not confused by normal cyclical changes in her breasts. She checks her cervical mucus to see whether she is fertile or not. She checks her genitalia once every six months, with her own disposable, personal-use speculum, flashlight, and mechanic's tiny mirror. She knows what her normal cervix looks like, because she has seen it with her own eyes. This woman is so body-informed that she even diagnosed one of her own pregnancies, by observing the bluish color change in her cervix during a self-exam. If anything is out of the ordinary, she is ready to deal with it. Sometimes, she only has to alter her diet or nutritional supplements to change a thick, bordering-on yeasty vaginal discharge into the normal, cleansing flow. At other times, she may seek out her midwife or doctor to discuss a change she has observed in her body, and perhaps have some diagnostic lab tests performed to help in discovering what is wrong.

Our naturally healthy woman appreciates the Creator who designed her, and enjoys her design. This understanding and enjoyment of her body benefits her husband, allowing him, as the Song of Solomon says, to enjoy fully the bounty of her garden.

We are all concerned about the serious health problems that can affect women. A woman engaged in informed Well WomanCare is more likely to catch those problems early, when treatments are not as harsh and mortality rates are not as high. That fact alone should be enough to make all of us want to be like that Naturally Healthy Woman.

C<small>HAPTER</small> 2

R<small>OUTINE</small> T<small>ESTING</small>

R<small>OUTINE</small> T<small>ESTING</small>

Most women do not look forward to the routine tests that are done each year or every two years in the gynecologist's office: pap smear, blood and urine tests, and possibly a mammogram after age forty, unless family history indicates the need for an earlier baseline mammogram. Either we become afraid of what the test results might tell us, or we simply do not want to deal with the procedures or physicians who do not respect our own beliefs or body instincts. In this section, we will explore the benefits of these tests as well as their risks, if any, so that we can decide individually what is best for us.

Basic Gynecological Examination

The basic gyn exam goes something like this: Ginger shows up for her appointment with her healthcare provider. (I will be using the term doctor in this example as most women see doctors for their well-woman care. This is not an indication that I think they are the only healthcare providers qualified to administer quality care. I have used midwives in my well-woman care where available in my area, and doctors as the need arose.) Ginger, we hope, does not have a long wait in the waiting room. Ideally, her healthcare provider has placed quality educational material throughout the room, in order for Ginger to make the best use of her time. When the nurse calls Ginger in to her examining room, she weighs Ginger, and takes her blood pressure. The nurse should take some time to write Ginger's concerns in her medical record, so that the doctor can have at least a clue about them when they meet.

The doctor, on greeting Ginger, should take some time to chat with her about what's going on in her life, any changes in normal body happenings, as well as any specific concerns Ginger might have about her health. If this is Ginger's first visit to the doctor, this exchange should occur in doctor's office or educational room. A woman should not have to meet a new doctor for the first time unclothed and on an examining table. If this happens to you, find another doctor.

After this exchange, Ginger is usually asked to change into a gown that opens in the front, and hop onto the examining table. She may be asked to provide a urine specimen while she is changing clothes. Dr. Respectful and Nurse Friendly leave the room to give Ginger privacy as she changes and urinates in the adjoining bathroom. Some doctors' offices do not have private bathrooms; in these cases, Ginger would more than likely be asked to give a urine specimen prior to settling into her examining room.

After Ginger has donned her fashion-designer examining gown, and is seated on the examining table, Dr. Respectful will knock on the door, and come in with Nurse Friendly after receiving an "okay" from Ginger. Dr. Respectful will then ask Ginger to lie back with her head on the pillow. He should ask her about her monthly breast exams while he guides her through his performance of a thorough breast exam, which includes the axillary (underarm) area. After ascertaining that all is well in Ginger's breast, Dr. R will palpate Ginger's upper and lower abdomen to distinguish any areas of soreness or pain.

The Internal Exam

At this point, Dr. Respectful may ask Ginger to slide down to the far end of the table, so that her bottom is slightly over the end of the table. On the other hand, he may simply have Ginger draw her feet up onto the table, slightly apart, and let her legs flop apart at the knees. A doctor can do the internal exam in either of these positions with accuracy. While most doctors give women a sheet to drape over their gown, this is not necessary for an accurate exam and should be optional. Ginger, or you, may prefer to see what's going on. If Dr. Respectful is also Dr. Nice, she/he will have warmed her/his hands under warm running water before performing any examination, and will explain each part of the exam. It should go something like this:

Dr. Respectful: Ginger, I'm going to be touching your outer labia and inserting my fingers into the vagina now. (At this point, Dr. Respectful will also be doing an external visual exam of Ginger's external genital area.)

Ginger: Okay. (Ginger should feel the freedom to speak up if any part of the exam is uncomfortable to her. It's not unheard of to get pubic hair pulled or delicate skin pinched accidentally during this procedure. Feel free to express your discomfort—kindly.)

At this point, Dr. Respectful will do what is termed a "bimanual palpation of the uterus, fallopian tubes and ovaries." What that means is that one of the doctor's hands will be on Ginger's lower abdomen, and one to two of the doctor's fingers will be touching the cervix inside Ginger's vagina. This helps the doctor feel the position, size and shape of Ginger's uterus, whether it is mobile or fixed, detect any pain and ascertain if there are any unusual growths on the uterus, tubes or ovaries. Obesity may make a bimanual exam difficult, but not impossible. Ginger's job is to concentrate on relaxing, and telling her doctor about any sensations she feels that are noteworthy: "That stings." "Ouch. That area sure is sore." "That side feels different from the other side you checked." Every detail Ginger can provide will help the doctor give Ginger a more accurate diagnosis if there is a problem.

Dr. Respectful will also do a rectal examination of Ginger after the bimanual exam. This is to determine the relative health of the posterior (back side) surfaces of the uterus and broad ligaments, the uterosacral ligaments, the posterior cul-de-sac and the structures on the lateral pelvic walls. A rectocele (where the wall of the rectum is protruding into the vaginal vault) and lower bowel lesions, such as polyps or tumors, can also be felt. This may be slightly uncomfortable, as the pressure exerted on the rectum during the exam feels a bit like the need to have a bowel movement. I can recall a visit with my own physician years ago when he felt the need to do a rectal exam. I said, "Oh, great. I really love this part," in a rather sarcastic tone of voice. His rapid reply was joined with a grin, "Well, it's not exactly the favorite part of my day, either." This still makes me chuckle.

After these manual examinations, the doctor will definitely ask Ginger to "scoot her bottom down to the end of the table." Warm, flannel stirrup pads will thoughtfully have been provided, for Ginger to place her feet in during the exam. She will allow her legs to relax apart. Dr. R, gently and slowly (while telling Ginger what will happen next), will insert a warmed speculum (an instrument that looks a bit like an alligator's snout, that is closed when inserted, then jacked open, allowing the doctor to see the vaginal vault and cervical area, and to insert the Pap smear sampling device) into the vaginal vault. The doctor will then direct the light so that a visual examination of the vaginal walls and cervix may be conducted. And last, but not least, the Pap smear will be obtained.

Most women who feel some discomfort during this exam do so during the insertion of the speculum. This may be due to a cold speculum. Why any doctor would think that anyone would want a cold metal instrument inserted into a body orifice is quite beyond me! Warming the speculum under warm running water, or using a plastic, disposable speculum, is much kinder and more comfortable. The discomfort may also come from a doctor who uses a speculum that is too large for a small woman's vagina. Ask for a smaller instrument. You pay the bills; you are the one uncomfortable. A simple, "That seems a bit large. Do you have a smaller size?" could make you not dread the next year's visit. And, certainly, if Dr. Respectful is being a bit rough in the exam, it is entirely appropriate to say, "That feels a bit rough. Could you be more gentle?"

One of the hardest things for a woman to do in her doctor's office is speak up and voice her opinions about the way she feels or the way she would like to be treated. This is sad. We have indoctrinated an entire generation or two of women who believe so strongly that doctor always knows best that they will endure cold attitudes, cold stirrups, cold hands, cold speculums, and an unhealthy doctor-patient relationship, rather than voice their preferences, which could help make for more comfort and a more respectful relationship for all women. Voicing one's feelings and preferences does not make one a militant feminist. It makes you a woman who understands that she is an important part of a successful physician's practice and that, as a woman informed about how her own body functions and its normal behavior, she is a vital portion of good diagnoses and health care.

THE PAP SMEAR

The Pap smear, a screening tool for detecting abnormal cells or suspicious cells that could develop into cancer and abnormalities in the cervix, is one of the most successful cancer screening tools developed. The test was developed by Dr. George Papanicolaou in the 1940s. Deaths from cervical cancer in women have been reduced by approximately seventy percent (that drop occurred between 1950 and 1970). Many women who might not have been diagnosed until their cervical cancer had grown significantly and spread have been able to engage in early intervention techniques that have literally saved their lives.

Pap smears are usually performed by having a physician or midwife gently scrape cells from the cervix and place them on a slide for a pathologist or cytologist to examine under a microscope for suspicious or abnormal cells. The cells that are scraped off are those that are already being sloughed off; the doctor is not taking a living layer of your skin off. The screening test is not one hundred percent accurate. False negatives may occur, when there is actually an abnormality on the cervix, or a false positive may occur, when there is no abnormality on the cervix. This is uncommon. Less than one percent of Pap smears are reported as false negative.

Physicians and midwives generally recommend that three annual Pap smears should be performed initially. After that, smears can be performed less than once a year if a patient is low risk. The sad result of the so-called "free love" generation is that few women qualify as low risk, which means no more than two lifetime sexual partners, and a partner with no more than two lifetime partners. Thus, many women should continue to have a yearly Pap smear; after sixty-five, all women should have an annual exam.

When Can a False Negative Occur?

The physician or midwife may not have been able to reach the area of abnormality with the sampling device, or the cells may not have been transferred from the sampling device to the slide. Sometimes, the abnormal cells are so small that the laboratory could not see them. At other times, the abnormal cells may be seen as normal by the laboratory personnel. Most laboratories that evaluate Pap smears do many, many Pap smears daily. Human error is not unheard of, even though it may not be common. Since cervical cancer usually progresses quite slowly, the best way to protect ourselves from false negatives is to have at least a yearly Pap smear, and possibly to choose some of the newer Pap technology, such as the ThinPrep® or computers to recheck Pap smears.

Thin Prep®

The thin-layer technology, that is used by Thin Prep® by CyTyc, involves collecting the cervical sample and putting the sample into a bottle of liquid instead of smearing the cells on a glass slide as is done during a regular Pap smear. The bottle is sent to a laboratory where a processor deposits a thin layer of cells onto a slide. This type of preparation may increase the likelihood that any abnormal cells will be transferred from the cervix to the slide. Another aspect of Thin Prep® is that, instead of the standard instrument used to scrape cells from the cervix, a brush-type of collection instrument is used, which may increase the chance that any area of abnormality on the cervix will be adequately scraped and the cells transferred to the collection bottle. The disadvantage to the Thin Prep® is that it does cost slightly more than the standard Pap smear, and may not be available in all doctors' offices. I had to travel ninety miles in order to get a Thin Prep® Pap test done after the standard test came back with inflammatory cells present.

Pap Smear Re-Check Technology

All laboratories are required to recheck at least 10% of all negative or normal Pap smears. This is part of their quality control procedures. A woman always has the right to request a re-screen of her Pap smear by the cytopathology laboratory personnel in the lab her Pap was sent to.

A woman may also decide to avail herself of one of the two FDA-approved computer-assisted devices for rechecking: "AutoPap," made by NeoPath in Redmond, Washington, and "PAPNET," made by Neuromedical Systems in Suffern, New York. AutoPap labs conduct Pap smear re-screening on site. After a woman's Pap smear slide has been screened and rated negative or normal, the AutoPap instrument rates the slide for the possibility of abnormal cells. If the rating indicates possible abnormal cells, the slide is rechecked by laboratory cytopathologists. The PAPNET system works in the same way, except the woman's Pap smear slide is sent to Neuromedical Systems' facility in New York to be rechecked. The PAPNET system creates digitized video images of the suspicious cells, and sends them back to the originating, local laboratory. The pictures are then reviewed on a computer screen by the cytopathologists. Studies have used PAPNET re-screening to reexamine previous negative pap smears taken from women with high-grade cervical cell abnormalities or cervical cancers. These studies found that in about one-third of these women, PAPNET testing detected abnormalities missed by manual screening on previous Pap smears.

Women at Highest Risk for Cervical Cancer have or have had:

1. No Pap smear
2. Infrequent Pap smears
3. Multiple sexual partners
4. Intercourse before age 18
5. Used oral contraceptives
6. Mother took the estrogen-like drug diethylstilbestrol (DES) during pregnancy to prevent miscarriage (common practice between 1940 and 1970)
7. Smoked cigarettes
8. Compromised immune system (AIDS or cancer)
9. Sexual partners who:
   a) have genital warts caused by HPV (Human Papilloma Virus)
   b) have had multiple sexual partners

How Can I Assure the Most Accurate Pap Smear Result Possible?

1. Schedule your gynecologic exam at the optimum time—two weeks after the first day of your last menstrual period. Do not schedule it during your menstrual period. If your gyn appointment was made months in advance, as most are these days, you will want to call the office to reschedule as soon as you work out that it will fall during your menstrual period.
2. Do not use vaginal medications, creams, tampons, contraceptives, or douches for 72 hours (3 days) prior to the exam.
3. Abstain from intercourse for 24 hours before the exam. Semen makes the slide difficult to read with any great deal of accuracy.
4. Make sure your Pap smear is sent to an accredited laboratory that employs nationally-certified cytotechnologists and board-certified pathologists. A little homework goes a long way here!
5. Call your doctor to get your test results and schedule any follow-up necessary. Do not depend upon your doctor's office to call you with test results, even if they tell you not to call. It's your body and your life at stake—make the call. If the test came back inconclusive, or with cells the doctor does not consider a risk, make a follow-up visit with the doctor or with another, particularly if you have a family history of cervical cancer or are in a high-risk category.

Unsatisfactory Pap smear

Some women get a call from the doctor's office with the nurse saying that the woman's Pap smear was "unsatisfactory," or that lab personnel were "unable to read results." What does this mean? There can be many reasons why a Pap smear may be read as "unsatisfactory" or have been unable to be read. A thick, but normal, vaginal secretion, or, more commonly, a cervical or vaginal infection, will give you inflammation. Some of the internal cervical cells may not have been collected on the slide. Rarely, a menstrual period may result in too many blood cells and not enough epithelial (cervical wall) cells to assess. Any of these circumstances may result in the cytopathologist being unable to read the results accurately; thus, we may get a call to come in for a repeat test. This does not mean your Pap smear was abnormal. It just needs to be rechecked to obtain an accurate result.

Abnormal Pap Results

There are varying degrees of "abnormal" on a Pap test. Since all of them are termed "cervical dysplasia," we will address abnormal Pap smears in Part Five, Chapter 3: Cervical Dysplasia.

Do I Need a Pap After a Hysterectomy?

We really have not definitive agreement among the medical community as to whether women who have had a hysterectomy continue to need Pap smears. Some folks say never; other folks say once every three to five years. A recent study[1] looked at the frequency of abnormal Pap smears in women who have had a hysterectomy. Their study was conducted in women over fifty, of whom twenty-five percent had had a hysterectomy. The researchers estimate that about forty-four to fifty percent of women in the U.S. who have had hysterectomies continued to have regular Pap smears. As they studied 21,152 of these post-fifty years of age women, those who had hysterectomies only had abnormal Pap smears 1.7 times out of 1,000. Another study at a university clinic that followed women who had hysterectomies over an average of fourteen years found an abnormal Pap rate of 3.5/1000. Even very high-risk women with hysterectomies were only found to have an abnormal Pap rate of 14.7/1000, which is close to that of the normal population with uteri in place.

Now, you are probably asking the same question I asked my own mother when she told me last year she needed to go in for her Pap smear (she had a hysterectomy when she was thirty, because of uterine cancer): How can a woman who has had a hysterectomy have a Pap smear, let alone an abnormal one? The medical truth is that the changes in the epithelium that take place on the cervix to produce abnormal Pap smears can also take place at the end of the vagina. So, post-hysterectomy, the physician is actually scraping the end of the vagina's epithelial cells during a Pap smear. Vaginal dysplasia, just like cervical dysplasia, may also develop, particularly in women who have previously had cervical dysplasia or cancer. Any woman who had a hysterectomy due to cervical dysplasia or cervical cancer should have yearly Pap smear screenings of her upper vaginal vault.

Treatment for vaginal dysplasia is the same as for cervical dysplasia, and is discussed in that section of this book.

The Bottom Line (!) on Pap Smears:

The test itself does not place a woman at higher risk for disease conditions, so I believe it quite prudent to find a good supportive midwife who does well-woman care, or a doctor, and get those yearly Paps. Women at high risk for cervical cancer should definitely consider having either a Thin Prep® Pap test or one of the computer re-checking programs.

YEARLY BLOOD AND URINE TESTS

Generally, the yearly blood and urine tests performed during a well-woman care visit are to evaluate basic health. Yes, doctors and midwives know that we are unlikely to be in a doctor's office other than this one visit per year if we are generally healthy people, so they endeavor to ascertain as much information as possible about our general health.

The standard blood tests are to check:

- hemoglobin and hematocrit levels, which will clue your health care provider in to anemia, which may indicate the need for further tests if symptoms are of excessive blood loss with menstruation or pain that could be associated with internal bleeding;
- white blood cell counts, if infection is suspected, such as when unexplained pelvic pain is present that needs to be differentiated between pelvic inflammatory disease (PID) and appendicitis or between tubal pregnancy and acute fallopian-tube or ovarian infection;
- thyroid function tests may be performed if symptoms warrant further investigation, particularly in women over 30.
- Blood tests are done by taking blood from a vein in your arm. Pain is minimal. Be certain to apply good pressure to the tiny wound prick after withdrawal of the needle, so that uncomfortable bruising does not occur.

Urine Tests

The urine examination is helpful since urinary tract infections occur fairly frequently in women. Sometimes, a woman will have no symptoms, yet she will have an underlying case of cystitis (bladder infection). This test is not invasive in the least; you only have to urinate into a cup. It is generally best to write your name on the label or directly on the cup prior to urinating into it. Your results will be more accurate if you clean your vaginal area with a wet paper towel prior to voiding into the cup.

Cultures

If a vaginal, cervical or pelvic infection is suspected, a culture may be done at the yearly visit. This is generally recommended if a woman has been experiencing heavy vaginal discharge and/or having abdominal pain or pain in her cervix. The doctor will cleanse the outer vaginal area with a long cotton swab, so that the culture from further up in the vaginal vault may be more accurate. Cultures aid in the diagnosis of vaginitis, either candidiasis, non-specific bacterial vaginosis or trichomoniasis, gonorrhea or chlamydia. An early diagnosis of gonorrhea or chlamydia is especially important due to the risk of infertility from these sexually-transmitted diseases.

A mammogram is a low-dose x-ray picture of the breast. The x-ray can find small breast cancer lumps that cannot be felt during a self-exam. This is especially important when one considers that by the time a tumor is perceptible, radiation and chemotherapy may be necessary in addition to either lumpectomy or mastectomy to prevent further growth of a cancerous tumor. There are two kinds of mammograms: a screening mammogram and a diagnostic mammogram.

Screening mammograms are those that most women have when they go in for a baseline mammogram at forty (or before if there is a family history of early onset breast cancer) and those having yearly mammograms who have had no previous history of breast tumors in family or self. Two x-ray pictures are taken of each breast. A trained radiologic technician will place the woman's breast on the mammogram machine where the breast will be compressed flat, then the technician will turn the "paddles" sideways for a side compression and view of the breast. A radiologist will look at the x-rays to decide if there is a problem needing further diagnostic testing.

Diagnostic mammograms are used if there is a breast problem. Perhaps the radiologist saw something in the screening mammogram that needs further investigation or maybe the woman had found a "lump" in her breast. This type of mammogram may be more time intensive and more pictures may be taken to ensure that the area of concern is in the picture. The radiologist will check the x-rays while you wait. Diagnostic mammograms are also used routinely for women with breast implants and women whose history or circumstances makes the doctor feel it necessary.

When Should I Have My First Mammogram?

Most health care providers are now recommending that women have a baseline mammogram done around age forty. Women with a maternal family history of breast cancer or repeated breast problems should have their baseline earlier. For me, because my mother had tumors removed in her early thirties as did my grandmother, who had half a breast removed, I chose to begin my mammogram screening in my early thirties.

The general recommendations primarily state that women fifty or over need to have a mammogram at least once every two years. The American Medical Association and the American Cancer Society both recommend that women forty and over have annual screening mammograms. While a baseline may be done at an earlier age, breast tissue looks different in premenopausal women, and may obscure an accurate result, particularly if the woman is breastfeeding. Early detection is a key to treating breast cancer effectively.

What Happens When I Go For My Mammogram?

While getting ready for your appointment, do not apply deodorant or antiperspirant to your underarms, as this may obscure x-ray findings. If you have forgotten, or if your appointment is later in the day, you will be provided with a cleansing cloth to clean off the deodorant/ antiperspirant residue. The technologist will give you a gown to wear, that opens in the front. She will position you in front of a special x-ray machine and place your breast on a plate that holds the x-ray film. This plate may be lowered or raised to match your height. A second plate will slowly be pushed down to make the breast flat. The technologist will position your arms and hands on the machine, or holding back your other breast, so that a full picture of your breast can be taken with the lowest dose of radiation possible. There is some pressure to the breast while the x-ray picture is being taken, but it is not painful, unless you have had previous breast surgery, or some soreness related to menstrual cycle changes. I have found the most difficult part is the feeling of playing twister when my arms and hands are being placed here and there.

My first mammogram was difficult. I knew I should have one, but I really didn't want to be there. I wanted to keep living my life without worrying about the specter of breast cancer. I was also wary because of my dislike of new situations, and having my breasts exposed to someone I didn't know. The technologist was very kind to me. She didn't ogle my breasts, although she did have to touch them for proper placement. After I was able to relax, I thought to myself: "Why have I been worrying over another woman catching a glimpse of my breast, or touching them, for a test, when I readily shed my gowns during labor without a care for what anybody thinks?"

To prepare for your mammogram:

1. Stop drinking caffeinated drinks several days before your mammogram appointment.
2. If you are still having periods, schedule your mammogram for the week after your period. Your breasts will be less tender and have fewer lumps. (This is also the best time to perform breast self-examination.)
3. If you take hormones (estrogen and progesterone), ask your doctor about the best time to schedule a mammogram.
4. If breast pain is a problem for you, you may consider using a pain reliever such as acetaminophen (Tylenol) or ibuprofen (Advil or Motrin) one or two hours before your

mammogram. Although this is a general recommendation from mammography centers, I truly believe it to be unnecessary.

It is best to refrain from using deodorant and powder on the day of your mammogram. These products contain metallic bases and may cause specks on your mammogram. Talk with the technologist performing your exam if you are concerned about the discomfort of a mammogram. She will apply compression slowly and only to a level that is tolerable for you.

What Happens After My Mammogram?

You will receive a card in the mail, or your physician may call you, if your results are normal. If there is a need for follow-up, your card will indicate that and you will definitely receive a call from your physician's office, telling you of the radiologist's concern. Most of the time, the radiologist will only recommend that a follow-up mammogram be done in six months to a year. If there is anything suspicious, more diagnostic testing will be initiated. If you have been told you have a tumor but that it is not believed to be cancerous, and you still have concerns or have other symptoms of breast cancer, do not hesitate to get another mammogram, diagnostic ultrasound or a second radiologist's opinion. It's your body; it's your life!

Concerns Regarding Mammograms

Q: I really believe that the radiation over time builds up and damages the health of my body, making me more susceptible to breast cancer. Isn't the very thing they are using for early diagnosis causing the disease they're trying to prevent?

A: I used to believe this completely. I was very concerned about low-dose radiation over the long term. My best friend in high school's dad was an x-ray technologist, and I can remember the radiation meter he wore on his clothes every day to work to check how much radiation he was receiving. Buildup is definitely a concern; however, when I really began to investigate how much radiation we receive from a mammogram, I was astounded. We receive more radiation from one cross-country flight in an airplane than during a routine mammogram, about as much also as standing on top of a mountain in Colorado. Now, I'm unwilling to cut out the convenience of airplanes for cross-country trips, and even though I don't want to stand on top of a mountain in Colorado, lots of other women would. Will I choose to ignore an early detection procedure that could help keep me around to enjoy my growing children, when it is no more risky than my flight up to Seattle, Washington?

Q: I'm a premenopausal woman who has been pregnant and breastfeeding for…well, the last 20 years. Do I really need a mammogram when I began having children early, have had six children, and breastfed each one and have no other risk factors?

A: The concern about premenopausal women having mammograms is that they have denser breasts, making it difficult to distinguish on mammograms harmless tissue from malignant tumors. A low-risk woman, who is being very thorough in her monthly self-exams and has worked to lower her breast cancer risk through diet, exercise, childbearing and breastfeeding, may be able to follow many scientists' recommendations and wait until fifty to start being screened. This is a personal decision. It has to be made with the risks in mind versus the benefit of the diagnostic procedure. Although breast cancer is uncommon in women under fifty, the age of breast cancer onset is lowering. Current statistics tell us that, of all women forty to forty-nine, only sixteen in every thousand will be diagnosed with breast cancer. In contrast, about seventy of every thousand will get be diagnosed between the ages of sixty to seventy-nine.

Why Can't I Just Do Breast Exams?

Only one study out of Canada supports the diligent breast exam alternative to mammograms, and it has been highly questioned by most medical authorities. Dr. Cornelia J. Baines of the University of Toronto, coauthor of the study which appeared in the Journal of the National Cancer Institute, says: "The study shows that women who are unable or unwilling to get mammograms can protect themselves equally well from breast cancer death by getting thorough annual physical breast examinations." In the Toronto study, 39,405 women volunteers, aged fifty to fifty-nine, were divided into two groups—one that periodically received both mammography and careful physical examinations, and a second group that received physical examinations only. Both groups were trained in breast self-examination, but Dr. Baines said it is not clear if this played a role in the results. The patients were enrolled between 1980 and 1985, and were followed for an average of thirteen years. By the end of 1993, the different screening techniques had detected about an equal amount of cancer. There were 622 invasive tumors and 72 in-place tumors in the mammography group, and 610 invasive tumors and 16 in-place tumors in the physical exam-only group.

The number of breast cancer deaths also was nearly equal: 107 for the mammography group and 105 deaths in the other group. The study results led Dr. Baines to say, that "the addition of annual mammography screening to physical examination has no impact on breast cancer survival." However, Baines did note that all the patients in the study received highly competent physical breast examinations. "The quality of the examination in our study is better than that generally found in medical practices," she acknowledged.[2] "If you happen to be among those women who can't afford mammography or don't like it and the pain and tenderness associated with it, go get a good clinical breast cancer physical exam and you will be protecting yourself against breast cancer death." Dr. Baines also clearly said that she was not advocating abandoning mammography screening.

Dr. Robert A. Smith, director of cancer screening at the American Cancer Society, says, "The advantage of mammography is that it finds small tumors." Certainly, not one of us could argue that it is better to have later detection with more radical therapy for breast cancer. Early breast cancer detection may mean that the cancer can be treated with even a small incision to remove the lump and no further chemotherapy or radiation necessary.

The primary concern with a woman doing her own breast self exams, or even having her obstetrician/gynecologist do a yearly exam, is that neither may give the quality of exam necessary to detect early cancer. I was unable to feel my own breast tumor, found early in 2000, and my doctor, who was very thorough, was unable to detect the tumor, even after we had both seen the thing on the x-ray picture and diagnostic ultrasound. The surgeon was the only one of us to actually feel the tumor before my surgery. I am pleased to say that, even with all the whirlwind of concern that tumor created, it turned out to be benign.

Is There Clear Evidence That Supports Mammograms?

Screening mammograms in women over forty reduces breast cancer deaths by fifteen percent, according to a study published in the International Journal of Cancer, and, clearly, regular mammograms reduce breast cancer deaths in women from fifty to sixty-nine by about a third. One major concern of those fighting breast cancer is that breast tumors appear to be faster growing in younger women, an observation cited as evidence by each side of the debate over routine mammograms for those forty to forty-nine, though these women have better survival rates than their older counterparts. In the clinical trials analyzed in the cancer journal, intervals between screening ranged from one year to three years. The death rate might even be cut further than fifteen percent if every woman in her forties had annual mammograms, the journal article concluded.

Many of the cancers detected by mammography in women under fifty are confined to a milk duct and are not invasive. Some scientists have questioned whether this type of tumor, known as ductal carcinoma in situ, or DCIS, is really cancer. Not all DCIS evolves into invasive cancer, but determining whether it will progress is tricky, if not impossible, given the current state of knowledge. "This represents a real clinical challenge," says Robert Smith, senior director in the cancer society's cancer control department. "But to suggest that DCIS is not a lesion that must be taken seriously is really not borne out by the data."

While there may still be some debate over the necessity of mammograms for a woman in her forties, we still have a clear indication that women over fifty definitely should be screened regularly. If so much of our Naturally Healthy lives are taken up with preventive measures, it would seem wise to add yearly mammograms to our prevention routine.

Chapter 3
Self-Examinations

One of the most important self-exams a woman can do each month is the Breast Self Exam or BSE. The guidelines for doing a BSE are below, provided by the Susan G. Komen Breast Cancer Foundation, September 2000.

At the same time each month, check for any changes in the normal look or feel of your breasts. Look for a lump, hard knot, or skin that thickens or dimples. Report any changes to your doctor or nurse. Go for regular breast exams and Pap tests. Ask about a mammogram.

Check your breasts using these steps:

Lying down:
Place a pillow under your right shoulder. Put your right hand under your head. Check your entire breast area with the finger pads of your left hand. Use small circles and follow an up-and-down pattern. Use light, medium, and firm pressure over each area of your breast. Gently squeeze the nipple for any discharge. Repeat these steps on your left breast.

Before a mirror:
Check for any changes in the shape or look of your breasts. Note any skin or nipple changes such as dimpling or nipple discharge. Inspect your breasts in four steps: arms at sides, arms overhead, hands on hips pressing firmly to flex chest muscles, and bending forward.

In the shower:
Raise your right arm. With soapy hands and fingers flat, check your right breast. Use the same small circles and up-and-down pattern described above in "Lying Down." Repeat on your left breast.

Inspection of moles and other skin growths:

It is also important to keep a check on your moles and other skin growths. Remember periodically to look over your body and notice whether there has been a change in the size, shape, color or texture of your moles. See your physician if you observe any of the following:

- A mole has developed a lighter colored halo or ring around it;
- The edges of the mole are not symmetrical, i.e. a nice, round mole has become ragged-edged;
- A mole has grown, particularly if it is over the size of a pencil eraser (about ¼ inch);
- The color of the mole has grown darker, even if only in one part of the mole;
- The mole feels rough or scaly;
- The mole bleeds when you touch it.

CHAPTER 4
HOW TO READ YOUR MEDICAL RECORD

WHY IT IS IMPORTANT TO KEEP YOUR OWN RECORDS:

My husband, who works for a hospital, told me about how hospitals discourage patients from requesting their medical records. The records are never offered to a patient. Often, when we request our records, we are asked why we want them, as if that should matter, asked to pay an exorbitant fee for them (friends recently told me about being charged $350 for their daughter's birth and NICU records), or informed that we need a medical professional with us when we read them because we simply will not be able to understand them. Well, I may not understand all the terminology when I sit down to read, but this is my health that is being chronicled, and I want to know what is being said. And I do know how to use a dictionary!

There are important reasons for keeping accurate records at home as well as at the hospital. Those records can save your life. For instance, if you do not know what you are allergic to, you could receive the wrong medication. All allergic reactions are not placed in medical records. I had a severe reaction to succinylcholine during surgery in 1999. That fact is not in my records. I did keep that information written down, and I place it on all medical record sheets that I have to fill out. I even place bold asterisks around my drug allergy information, because I have been treated by doctors who tried repeatedly to give me medications to which I am allergic. In our own home records, we keep a log of illnesses, medications taken and any reactions to those medications, and notes from visits to doctors and midwives, including what was tested, discussed and diagnosed.

It is helpful to take your log with you every time you visit a doctor or hospital. If you can, take along a friend as well. She can witness what goes on, and serve as a listening ear in case you miss hearing something that is important to your health. These two actions help prevent errors from occurring. According to my husband, they are all too frequent for us to ignore the possibility. Many doctors find it intimidating to have another person in the room with the patient; they know they are going to be accountable. This is a good situation. You might say it evens things up, because most patients feel intimidated by the mere fact that they are in a doctor's (expert's) office. My mother taught me very early that one should never see a doctor alone, or stay even a minute in the hospital alone. Years ago, I thought her advice a bit odd. Now, I see her incredible wisdom. Even the strongest of women usually feels intimidated by doctors and hospitals. My mother has nursed so many of our family through illnesses, and now I try to go with her when she needs medical attention, to serve as her advocate. Remember: The Naturally Healthy Woman not only looks after and respects her divinely designed body, she also insists that professional caregivers give her the same respect.

Keeping your own medical records:

Your first step is to obtain your existing medical records. The best way to do this is to make a list of all the doctors you have seen, beginning with the most recent, as well as all the hospitals in which you have been treated. Look up the addresses and telephone numbers, if available. If you have internet access, you can find them through the online yellow pages. Once you have these, write to each doctor and hospital, explaining that you are trying to establish a home medical record that will

● serve as a family history for your children;
● help you as you continue to a) receive medical care, by putting you in a better position to provide important health information for future medical visits and b) work on disease prevention.

Always state in your letters: "I need full and complete copies of my entire medical record, to include all laboratory results, doctor's and nurse's notes, and any other diagnostic test results." Include all your pertinent identifying information: name, date of birth, SSN, and account numbers for that medical office or hospital. It helps to send in a check with your request—not three hundred and fifty dollars, which is a ridiculous figure to be expected to pay for your own medical records, but a reasonable amount—fifteen to twenty-five dollars—to cover copying charges and the time of the worker who will be doing the copying. Be polite and grateful in your letters for the time the doctor's office or hospital workers will take to copy your information and send it to you. Follow up with another letter, then a phone call, if you do not receive your records within one month's time.

Once you have your records in hand, the key to reading them is understanding the abbreviations commonly used by health care personnel:

a	= before
aa	= of each
a.c.	= before meals
ad	= to, up to
ADL	= activities of daily living
ad lib	= as needed, as desired
AF	= auricular fibrillation
agit	= shake, stir
AMA	= against medical advice
Ap.	= appendicitis
Aq	= water
ASA	= acetylsalicylic acid, aspirin
ASAP	= as soon as possible, urgent
ASCVD	= atherosclerotic cardiovascular disease
ASHD	= atherosclerotic heart disease
BE	= barium enema
b.i.d.	= twice a day
BKA	= below knee amputation
Bl. Time	= bleeding time
BM	= bowel movement
BMR	= basal metabolic rate
BP	= blood pressure
BPH	= benign prostatic hypertrophy, enlarged prostate
BRP	= bathroom privileges
BUN	= blood urea nitrogen
Bx	= biopsy
C.	= centigrade
c	= with
C1	= first cervical vertebrae
CA, Ca	= cancer
CAD	= coronary artery disease
cap(s)	= capsule(s)
CBC	= complete blood count
CBD	= common bile duct
CC	= chief complaint

cc	= cubic centimeter
CCU	= coronary care unit
CHD	= coronary heart disease; or congenital heart disease
CHF	= congestive heart failure
Chol	= cholesterol
Cl. time	= clotting time
CN	= cranial nerve
CNS	= central nervous system
comp	= compound
cont rem	= continue the medicine
COPD	= chronic obstructive pulmonary disease
Cor	= heart
CRF	= chronic renal (kidney) failure
C&S	= culture & sensitivity, a culture used to look for bacteria causing an infection as well as to find out what antibiotics can treat it.
C-sect	= cesarean section
CSF	= cerebrospinal fluid
CV	= cardiovascular
CVA	= cerebrovascular accident
CVP	= central venous pressure
Cx	= cervix; culture
CXR	= chest x-ray
d	= give
D&C	= dilation and curettage
d/c; DC	= discontinue; discharge from hospital or care
dd in d	= from day to day
DDx	= differential diagnosis, a list of possible causes or diagnoses for symptoms
dec	= pour off
dexter	= the right
DIFF	= differential blood count, a test for the number and types of white blood cells in the blood
dil	= dilute
disp.	= dispense
div	= divide
DM	= diabetes mellitus
DOE	= dyspnea on exertion, shortness of breath on walking or going up stairs or incline

dos	= dose
DTR	= deep tendon thrombosis, phlebitis or blood clots in the vein
dur dolor	= while pain lasts
D/W	= dextrose in water
Dx	= diagnosis
EBL	= estimated blood loss, commonly reported during any surgery
ECG or EKG	= electrocardiogram
EEG	= electroencephalogram
emp	= as directed
ENT	= ear, nose and throat
EOM	= extraocular movement, eye movement
ER	= emergency room
ESR	= erythrocyte sedimentation rate
ETOH	= ethanol, alcohol; alcoholic (sometimes written EtOH)
F.	= Fahrenheit
FBS	= fasting blood sugar
Fe	= iron
febris	= fever
FH	= family history
F/U	= follow-up, future appointment, testing or treatment needed
Fx	= fracture
GA	= general anesthesia
garg	= gargle
GB	= gallbladder
GC	= gonorrhea
GI	= gastrointestinal
GL	= glaucoma
gm	= grams
gr	= grains
grad	= by degrees
gravida	= pregnancies
gtt	= drops
GTT	= glucose tolerance test
GU	= genitourinary
GYN	= gynecology
h	= hour
HASHD	= hypertensive arteriosclerotic heart disease
Hb or Hgb	= hemoglobin

HCT	= hematocrit
HEENT	= head, eyes, ears, nose, throat
H/H	= hemoglobin and hematocrit, tests for anemia
HHD	= hypertensive heart disease
H/O	= history of
HOB	= head of bed
H&P	= history and physical, written report by your doctor describing your medical history and physical examination
HPI	= history of present illness
HS/hs	= at bedtime, before retiring
HSV	= herpes simplex virus
HTN	= hypertension, high blood pressure
Hx	= history
ICU	= intensive care unit
I&D	= incision and drainage
IM	= intramuscular
I.M.	= infectious mononucleosis
I&O	= intake and output (measure of fluids going in and out of the body)
IPPB	= intermittent positive pressure breathing
ind	= daily
IV	= intravenous
IVP	= intravenous pyelogram
JVP	= jugular venous pressure, visible measure of the jugular vein pressure in the neck, if elevated, a sign of heart failure
L	= left
L2, L3	= second, third lumbar vertebrae
LPB	= low pack pain
liq	= liquid
LLE	= left lower extremity
LLQ	= left lower quadrant
LMP	= last menstrual period
LNMP	= last normal menstrual period
LP	= lumbar puncture
LUE	= left upper extremity
LUQ	= left upper extremity
LV	= left ventricle, the largest muscle or chamber of the heart that pumps blood into the aorta

LVH	= left ventricular hypertrophy, thickening of the left ventricle muscle typically from untreated high blood pressure
'lytes	= common blood electrolytes (Na – sodium, K-potassium, Cl – chloride, Co_2 = carbon dioxide)
m	= murmur
M	= mix
MCP	= metacarpophalangeal joints, the joints between the hands and fingers
Meg	= milliequivalents, a metric unit of measurement
m et n	= morning and night
mg	= milligrams
MI	= heart attack (myocardial infarction)
MOM	= milk of magnesia
mor. dict.	= in the manner directed
M.S.	= morphine sulfate
MTP	= metatarsophalangeal joints, the joints between the foot and toes
Na	= sodium
NAD	= no acute distress; no active disease
neg	= negative
NG	= nasogastric
NL	= normal
NKA or NKDA	= no known drug allergies
no.	= number
non rep; nr	= do not repeat
NPO/npo	= non per os (nothing by mouth)
NS	= normal saline
NSR	= normal heart rate (normal sinus rhythm)
N&V	= nausea and vomiting
O	= objective; doctor's description of physical and laboratory findings
O_2	= oxygen
o	= none
OBS	= organic brain syndrome, confusion, senility
O.D.	= right eye
o.d.	= once a day
O.L.	= left eye
OOB	= out of bed
O&P	= ova and parasites, commonly checked for in the stool of a person with diarrhea

OPD	= outpatient department
OR	= operating room
O.S.	= left eye
OT	= occupational therapy
OTC	= over-the-counter medications sold without a prescription
OU	= both eyes
P.	= after
P	= pulse or number of pulse or heartbeats in a minute
Para	= number of births
Path.	= pathology
p.c.	= after meals
PCN	= penicillin
PE	= physical examination; or pulmonary embolus
PERRLA	= pupils, equal, round, reactive to light and accommodation (far and near vision)
PFT	= pulmonary function test
PI	= present illness
pil	= pill
PMH	= past medical history
PND	= paroxysmal nocturnal dyspnea, waking up at night short of breath, indicative of heart failure
PO/po	= by mouth
Post.	= posterior
post-op	= postoperative; after the operation
PPD	= purified protein derivative, skin test for tuberculosis
ppd	= refers to number of packs of cigarettes smoked daily
PR	= pulse rate; or, rectally
pre-op	= before surgery
PRN/prn	= as needed, as often as necessary
Prog.	= prognosis
pt	= patient
PT	= physical therapy
PTA	= prior to admission
PTT	= partial thromboplastin time, a test of blood clotting, measure of the blood thinner effect of heparin
PUD	= peptic ulcer disease, stomach or duodenal ulcer
Px	= prognosis
q.	= every

qd	= every day
q.h.	= every hour (q. 2h. = every two hours)
q.i.d.	= four times a day
q. n.	= every night
q.o.d.	= every other day
q.s.	= proper amount; quantity sufficient
q.v.	= as much as desired
R	= right
rbc	= red blood cell
RBC	= red blood cell count
rep	= repeat
RHD	= rheumatic heart disease
RLQ	= right lower quadrant
R.N.	= registered nurse
ROM	= range of motion
ROS	= review of systems, review of all your symptoms and concerns from head to toe
RR	= respiratory rate; or recovery room
RSR	= regular sinus rhythm, same as NSR
RT	= radiation therapy
RTC	= return to clinic, date when advised to return to doctor's office for appointment
rub	= red
RUQ	= right upper quadrant
Rx	= prescription; or therapy
s	= without
S&A	= sugar and acetone (a urine test for diabetics)
SC	= subcutaneous
Scop.	= scopolamine
SH	= social history
SICU	= surgical intensive care unit
sig	= write, let it be imprinted
sing	= of each
SMA	= sequential multiple analyzer, blood chemistry check of multiple tests
SOB	= shortness of breath
sol	= solution
solv	= dissolve

SOP	= standard operating procedure
SOS	= can repeat in emergency
S/P,s/p	= status post, after or previous history of a surgery or medical condition
ss	= half
S&S	= signs and symptoms
SSE	= soapsuds enema
stat	= right away, immediately
STD	= sexually-transmitted disease
sub Q	= subcutaneous
suppos	= suppository
Sx	= symptoms
T&A	= tonsillectomy and adenoidectomy
tab	= tablet
TAT	= tetanus antitoxin
tere	= rub
TIA	= transient ischemic attack
TIBC	= total iron-binding capacity, measure of amount of blood proteins carrying iron
t.i.d.	= three times a day
tinc or tinct	= tincture
TMJ	= temporomandibular joint, the joint between the skull and the jawbone, a site of chronic pain or dysfunction
TPR	= temperature, pulse and respiration
TURP	= transurethral resection of prostate, surgical chipping away of the prostate gland through the urethra to relieve blockage
Tx/TX	= treatment
UGI	= upper GI series, barium x-ray of the esophagus, stomach and duodenum
ung	= ointment
URI	= upper respiratory infection
ut dict	= as directed
UTI	= urinary tract infection
VD	= venereal disease
VS	= vital signs
WBC	= white blood cell count
WC	= wheelchair
WNL	= within normal limits
wt.	= weight

X	= times
x	= except
YO	= year old
Z/D	= zero defects

Understanding your lab work results:

The results of lab work can be confusing, especially when there are clear indications that something is "high" or "low," yet our physician says everything is fine. We need to understand at least what the blood tests we have are checking for.

Printed test results usually come with columns that list what is being checked, the "Reference Range," which is the range of normal values for each blood component, and a notice indicating values that are "Out of Range." "Out of Range" notices are normally accompanied by "H" for "high" or "L" for "low."

Complete Blood Count (CBC) gives the total number of cells in your blood, as well as their size and shape, which determines their health:

❋ White Blood Cell Count (WBC) counts the total number of white blood cells. White blood cells fight infection, so an elevated number (doctors call this "leukocytosis") can be a sign that your body is fighting infection or has a chronic inflammation. A high WBC can also occur when you are under extreme stress, or can result from certain medications. Even the herb echinacea can cause a slightly elevated WBC within two hours after it is taken so, if you know you are going to have a CBC done, do not take your echinacea that morning. Otherwise, you might not have an accurate picture of what is going on in your body. If your white blood cell count is low, your doctor will investigate further to see if you have a blood disorder, or if any medications you are taking have caused faulty results. If your CBC is a concern, your doctor may order a CBC w/differential, which will count all the different white blood cells that your immune system produces to keep you healthy.

❋ Red Blood Cell Count (RBC) is the total number of red blood cells, which carry oxygen in your blood. This count gives your doctor an overall picture of the health of your RBCs.

❋ Hemoglobin (Hb or Hgb) measures whether your cells have adequate amounts of the protein that carries oxygen. If this number is low, you have anemia and will probably be advised to take an iron supplement. Most women have Hb levels in the range of 12 to 14; men are slightly higher at 14 to 16. Excessive iron levels have been associated with cancer, so do not take iron supplements unless necessary.

❋ Hematocrit (Hct) gives the percent ratio of red blood cells to total blood volume. If it is low, this again is a sign of anemia. A woman's hematocrit is usually about 36%, although this number can decrease around the 28th week of pregnancy, when blood volume has expanded tremendously, causing a dilution of red blood cells that may be seen as anemia. Men usually average 42%.

❋ Mean Corpuscular Volume (MCV) gives the size and shape of red blood cells. This is an important value to watch, as certain types of anemia or nutrient deficiencies can cause RBCs that are too small or the wrong shape.

- Platelet Count shows whether you have enough of the cells that cause your blood to clot properly.

Erythrocyte Sedimentation Rate (ESR or SED Rate): This test measures how quickly your red blood cells settle to the bottom of a tube during a one-hour period. An elevated value can signal severe anemia, an infection, chronic inflammation, and some cancers.

Blood Chemistry

Glucose (blood sugar) is a screening test used to check for diabetes (if your level is higher than 135) or hypoglycemia (if it's lower than 70).

Blood Urea Nitrogen (BUN) and Creatinine are tests that give a picture of how well your kidneys are functioning.

Sodium, Potassium and Chloride are blood salts, or electrolytes. If you have heart disease or high blood pressure, these numbers will be very important. They are measuring for dehydration of vital salts that help our body function.

Uric Acid is a waste product of all cells. High levels can signal kidney problems or a condition called "gout."

Albumin is a blood protein produced by our liver. A low count can be a sign of liver or kidney disease.

Globulin is a blood protein produced by our immune system. A high count can point to chronic inflammation, infection or blood disorders.

Calcium is a component of our blood that helps our body function normally. This is not a test for bone density. A high count is called "hypercalcemia" and can indicate a problem with our parathyroid gland, which can lead to kidney stones and low bone density.

Serum Glutamine Pyruvic Transaminase (SGPT) and Serum Glutamate Oxaloacetate Transaminase (SGOT) are enzymes, or proteins, that give an idea of how your liver is functioning, since they are primarily produced in the liver. SGOT is also produced by the red blood cells.

Lactate Dehydrogenase (LDH) is an enzyme produced by many cells of the body. An extremely high level will cause your doctor to want to investigate further to rule out a possible malignancy somewhere in your body.

Bilirubin is a chemical in bile that gives it the yellow color. When the bile duct from the liver to the intestine is blocked, the bilirubin count will be high. Gallstones are the most common blockage problem, but liver disease must be ruled out.

Gamma Glutamyl Transpeptidase (GGT) is another enzyme produced by the liver. Excessive weight or alcohol intake are the most common reasons for elevation. This enzyme level can also be elevated when there is a blockage of the bile duct and with liver disease.

Alkaline Phosphatase is yet another enzyme produced by the liver and bones. If it is high, your doctor will look at your GGT level to find the cause. If you have both elevated alkaline phosphatase and GGT levels, your liver is having problems.

Blood Fats

This test may also be called a "lipid profile."

Total Cholesterol is the sum of both the LDL and HDL levels in your blood. High total cholesterol levels are linked to cardiovascular disease. Levels that are too low are associated with a slightly higher incidence of leukemia. Under 200 is desirable. If yours is too low, add some fat back into your life – good fat, please!

High-Density Lipoprotein (HDL) is the "good cholesterol." The high density needs to be a high number, at least 30% of the total cholesterol level.

Low-Density Lipoprotein (LDL) is the "bad cholesterol." You want this number to be 130 or less, with an ideal number for those with cardiovascular disease under 100.

Triglycerides are a form of fat in the blood. This level rises after meals, which is the reason you have to fast before having your lipid profile test done. Elevated levels combined with high cholesterol increase our risk of cardiovascular disease.

Thyroid Function Tests
Thyroxine 3 (T_3) measures the amount of unsaturated thyroid binding globulin (TBG) in your blood. If the level is low, suspect hypothyroidism; if it is high, suspect hyperthyroidism.

Thyroxine 4 (T_4) measures the combined free and bound total thyroxine level in the blood. Low may indicate hypothyroidism; high may indicate hyperthyroidism.

Thyroid Stimulating Hormone (TSH) measures the amount of the hormone that regulates the release and storage of thyroid hormone. A high level may indicate hypothyroidism; a low level may indicate hyperthyroidism. Values that are borderline should be periodically re-checked due to some conditions of hypo and hyperthyroidism not always showing up in the standard blood tests.

Part Three:
Bountiful Blessings

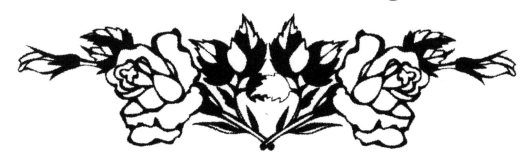

CHAPTER 1
HEALTHY PREGNANCY

Pregnancy and childbirth are spectacular times in a woman's life. Even though pregnancy is a normal part of life; it is a time filled with moments bordering on the miraculous: first knowledge that a new life is growing inside you; that first little tickle of movement; the first time a hand or foot pushes out on your skin, saying "hello." Then, after long months of waiting, comes the force of the contractions that will bring the baby into your arms, the glimpse of a head in the perineum that quickly turns into a whole, squirming little body gently laid upon your heart. Since The Naturally Healthy Pregnancy book covers pregnancy and childbirth in great detail, we will only address here the benefits of pregnancy, childbirth and breastfeeding in a woman's lifetime of health.

The Career of Motherhood

While our culture continues in its race toward further devaluation of life, we, as Christian women, know that children are a blessing from the Lord. We do not make the world's mistake of looking upon children as a burden, a chain preventing us from becoming who we want to be. We know that the gift of a child in our lives brings us great opportunities in our pursuit of holiness. Taking responsibility for our children helps us to relinquish our self-love and selfish ambition, allowing us to give this world what it truly needs: a growing people of God to expand Christ's kingdom and bring it to its fullness and glory on the earth.

Each day, throughout the day, my load is lightened by the joy my children bring, through their excited squeals as one chases another in tag, or as an old toy is rediscovered, with the dressing up of my little girls as they play house, and as the older ones come to me with stories of what they have just learned in a book they are reading. And I can think of no better way to end a day than to have ten or more arms reach out to me for bedtime hugs and kisses, with the shared murmurings of "I love you" and prayers that are so sweet and humble, yet so bold before the throne of God. Children are bountiful blessings indeed.

There is more, though, to pregnancy and childrearing than the joy and sanctification children bring into our lives. Pregnancy and breastfeeding confer some significant health benefits that should not be ignored. God has designed these conditions to be good for us. For instance, the risk of a woman developing all reproductive cancers is lowered if she begins childbearing and breastfeeding at an early age. The current cultural notion—that we should wait until our mid to late twenties before marrying, and then wait several more years before bearing children—is a step in an unhealthy direction. There is nothing wrong with a young woman who gets married and begins to bear children in her late teens, or early twenties. In fact, this may confer the greatest health benefit on young women.[1]

What about college? And a career? What about time just to "enjoy life?" Education, business dealings, enjoyment of life—these are all good things but, if they take precedence over a woman's primary calling, then there may be a problem in our basic thinking. Women were designed to be "helpmeets." It is hard to take on that function when we have not bothered to think about it until we have earned a degree, established a career, and had some fun. Only in the past and current generation have our ideas regarding the blessings of marriage and children changed so radically. Perhaps we should rethink how we prepare our daughters for their lives. And not only our daughters: we must train our sons carefully, teaching them to finish their education, and enter the work force early enough to establish a regular income that could support a wife and children.

A Fountain of Blessings

Breastfeeding confers significant reductions in breast cancer rates. Women who are breastfed as infants have a twenty-five percent reduction in the risk of developing breast cancer.[1] Breastfeeding for at least four to twelve months reduces a woman's risk by eleven percent. The incidence of breast cancer in premenopausal women is reduced by twenty-five percent if they have breastfed for twenty-four months. Women who bear no children are at higher risk for all reproductive cancers, as are those who bear their first child after age thirty. The benefits of breastfeeding may be greater if a woman becomes pregnant and lactates at an early age.[2]

Ovarian cancer rates also drop significantly in women having a fewer number of menstrual cycles throughout their lifetime. Therefore, the risk factors for ovarian cancer include: early onset of menses (before age twelve), late menopause (after age fifty), no pregnancies, or a first pregnancy after age thirty, and the use of fertility drugs, which induce ovulation and menstrual cycles. This means that a woman's overall risk of ovarian cancer is lowered the more children she has, combined with breastfeeding without supplemental infant formulas or rigid schedules. These prevent a baby from getting adequate nourishment, and a mother from gaining the benefit of breastfeeding amenorrhea for the thirteen-month average after birth.

A Case in Point: Ginger's Story

Let's look at a particular case: Ginger began menstruating when she was twelve, and had regular cycles every twenty-eight days. She married at age nineteen, and became pregnant right away. She was a knowledgeable breastfeeding mother, who knew that breast milk is metabolized in only one and a half to two hours, rather than the longer time it takes formulas to digest. Therefore, she gave her tiny infant night nursings, too, and breastfed for twenty-four months. This gave her fifteen months of no periods after the baby's birth.

Within a few months, she became pregnant again, and continued in that cycle of pregnancy followed by breastfeeding, with at most one year of cycles between pregnancies, for the next sixteen years. At that point, although she and her husband did not try to prevent pregnancy, she simply did not get pregnant again. Her cycles had become more irregular at age forty, and she began menopause around age forty-five. Ginger has always eaten well and exercised—taking care of her children kept her body young! Ginger has a very low risk of developing any of the reproductive cancers.

We may not all be like Ginger, but we can at least see the wisdom of God's design for protection of a woman's body in childbearing and breastfeeding. In our next two chapters, we will address the exceptions to Ginger.

Chapter 2
Infertility

The Lord God opens and closes the womb. However, we often engage in activities or habits that are not favorable for conception. We have a responsibility to steward our bodies, and to prepare them nutritionally for God to plant our husband's seed within us. Fathers also have a responsibility to make their bodies nutritionally ready to supply healthy seed. We must also recognize there are certain health conditions that may prevent pregnancy. Although we ultimately trust God to open the womb, I do feel that we are free to avail ourselves of natural and conventional medical technology, as long as that technology does not presume to "play god."

Following our Ladder Approach to Health Care™, we will address basic nutritional and lifestyle concerns first, then proceed to herbs and specific nutrients that may be helpful.

Basic Steps To a Healthy Reproductive System:

1. Follow the preconception care advice in Part One, Chapter 1: Pre-Puberty Health Care.
2. Some women may need to gain five or ten pounds if they are under their ideal weight. Women who exercise too much or are significantly underweight do not menstruate. If you are not menstruating, you are probably not ovulating. If you do not ovulate, you cannot get pregnant. Other women may need to lose weight. Body fat produces extra estrogen, which may create an estrogen-dominance syndrome that plays out like a progesterone deficiency, even though the woman may not be truly progesterone-deficient. Too much

body fat also creates a ripe environment for the development of Adult Onset (Type 2) Diabetes, which can reduce fertility, and compromise the health of an unborn baby.

3. Sperm perform best in a slightly acidic environment. Aid the body's slightly acidic vaginal environment by avoiding foods that contribute to a very alkaline environment: refined sugars, simple carbohydrates (starches) and alcohol. Sperm find it difficult to live in a very acidic environment; if the vagina is very acidic, a woman may want to douche with baking soda prior to intercourse, during her fertile days of the month. When she orgasms prior to her husband, she produces an alkaline discharge or fluid in the vagina that may work as well as the baking soda, without the inconvenience.

4. Keep a chart of the menstrual cycle for at least six months. If a woman ends up having to see a fertility specialist, she will need this chart anyway, to facilitate her treatment. There are two good books on how to chart menstrual cycles so that the fertile days of the month are easily recognized: The Art of Natural Family Planning by John and Sheila Kippley, and Taking Charge of Your Fertility by Toni Weschiler, M.P.H. This way, a couple can be sure that intercourse takes place during the fertile days. It is generally considered best to have intercourse once every two days during this time. And please, keep in mind that this is not supposed to be work. Whether you are "trying" for a baby or not, remember to enjoy one another. The knowledge that God is in control of this process, no matter how precisely we time our marital relations, can give us the peace necessary to delight in each other's body.

5. If cycles are irregular, follow the recommendations in Part One, Chapter 3: Cycle Regulation.

6. Have basic lab work done, and check additionally for normal thyroid and pituitary function. I do hasten to add that these tests are often unreliable for those on the edge of what is considered normal. A woman may need to visit a good reproductive endocrinologist if she feels she does have a problem that lab tests are not indicating. I have a good friend with Hashimoto's disease: her lab tests do not indicate a thyroid deficiency, yet her endocrinologist is able to see the subtle problems that her family physician completely missed.

7. Finally, don't allow becoming pregnant to become the focus of your life. Whether we are blessed with children or not, we still have many opportunities to minister to our local church body, our community, and the world around us. If we keep ourselves focused on our "going forth" each day with our daily tasks, we will be less likely to become obsessed with our lack of a child.

Nutritional supplement recommendations:

First, correct any deficiencies discovered through lab work. Herbal and vitamin supplements are a natural way to correct these deficiencies: they "feed" needed nutrients to the glands in a way that does not over-stimulate them. The following herbs have been shown in preliminary scientific investigations to help normalize the production of hormones by normalizing glandular function:

* Chaste berry (Vitex agnus-castus): German experiments and a German study showed that extracts of agnus-castus can stimulate the release of Leutenizing Hormone (LH) and inhibit the release of Follicle Stimulating Hormone (FSH). One other study suggested that the volatile oil has a progesterone-like effect.[1]

* False unicorn (Chamaelirium luteum): Current pharmacology indicates that the steroidal saponins have adaptogenic effect on ovaries (normalizing function).[2]

* Red raspberry (Rubus stringosus): Various species of red raspberry have been shown to induce ovulation as well as relax the uterus.[3]

* Wild yam (Dioscorea villosa): Wild yam is used as the basis of commercial birth-control products' sex hormone production (conversion of its steroid diosgenin to progesterone).[4] Although wild yam does not convert to progesterone in the human body, some herbalists believe it to be of benefit to those with low progesterone levels due to its effect on the adrenal glands as well as being beneficial for its antispasmodic effect on the uterus.

* Natural progesterone creme: Low progesterone levels in a woman's body do not allow the endometrial lining to build for the baby to implant and the pregnancy to be sustained. Mild cases of progesterone deficiency can probably be treated with the natural progesterone creme rather than progesterone suppositories. The exception would be the woman who has had repeated miscarriages. If a woman uses natural progesterone creme, she should make certain that it is not just a "wild yam" creme, as these contain no natural progesterone. The label needs to say natural progesterone and give the amount of progesterone delivered in each daily dose. She also should not use the creme except in the luteal phase of her cycle, after ovulation; otherwise, she will further cause imbalance with her hormones.

* Black Cohosh (Cimicifuga racemosa): Black Cohosh has estrogenic effects; that is, it acts like the female hormone estrogen, which makes it useful for those women with low estrogen levels.[5] Do not take after pregnancy is confirmed.

* Vitamin E deficiency is associated with low plasma levels of FSH and LH in pituitary tissue.[6]

* Panax and/or Siberian ginseng may be used for their adaptogenic effects on the body. Panax ginseng is contraindicated for pregnancy; therefore, potential mothers should not use Panax ginseng during the luteal phase of the cycle, when pregnancy may have already occurred. Sarsaparilla may also be used during the luteal phase for its purported progesteronic effect.

* Infertility due to scar tissue formation or endometriosis may require surgical intervention after careful weighing of the risks and benefits. An herbal therapy that may, or may not, help, is the application of castor oil packs. Soak a clean piece of flannel in 4 ounces of

castor oil. Warm it in the oven (be careful not to start an oven fire) and apply to the abdomen for 20 minutes to 1 hour daily for 2 weeks, or 2-3 times weekly for 6 weeks. Blue Cohosh and Black Cohosh stimulate tissue health of scarred structures when taken internally.[7]

Herb Formulas for Cycle Regulation:

B-Fruitful by TriLight Herbs is a formula I designed myself, for women needing herbs that support healthy hormonal function and balancing. The formula contains: False unicorn, vitex, Squaw Vine, True unicorn root, Black haw and ginger. Take ½ teaspoon 3 times daily throughout the menstrual cycle.

Lengthening the luteal phase (after ovulation until the bleeding begins): Vitex, once again, is the herb most used for this purpose. Vitex has a normalizing effect on the pituitary which controls the length of the luteal phase. As with all normalizing herbs, vitex may need to be taken several months to achieve results. 1-2 capsules of a standardized extract of vitex each morning is the usual dosage for cycle regulation purposes.

Basic Steps to Maximize Male Fertility:

1. Wear loose underpants and trousers. Do not sit in one place for long periods.
2. Do not sit in hot tubs.
3. Get adequate rest and regular exercise.
4. Nettles, oat straw and burdock may be added to men's daily routine for added nutrition.
5. Astragalus increased sperm motility when administered 10mg invitro.[8]
6. Studies have shown that nutrients are beneficial for improving sperm count and normal sperm formation.[9][10][11] The following supplement recommendations are based on empirical information as well as available scientific literature:
    - Arginine: 1.5-3 g daily for 3-6 months
    - Essential fatty acids provide the basis for prostaglandin production. Seminal fluid is rich in prostaglandins. Some men with low fertility of unknown origin have low levels of seminal prostaglandins.[12]
    - Zinc: 50 mg daily
    - Chromium: 50-200 mcg daily
    - Selenium: 50-100 mcg daily
    - Vitamin E: 400-600 IU daily for increased sperm motility and morbidity[13]
    - Vitamin A: 7500 IU daily
    - B Vitamins: 25 - 100 mg daily

- Vitamin C: 500 mg daily
- Free-form amino acids: 500 mg twice daily
- L-Lysine: 500 mg daily
- L-acetyl-L-carnitine: helps to increase sperm count and stimulate testosterone production[14]
- Glutathione: 600 mg daily, has shown significant benefits on sperm motility.[15]

Herbal Formula for Men #1:

Muira puama bark	1 oz
Panax ginseng root	3 oz
Siberian ginseng root	2 oz
Damiana herb	2 oz
Spearmint or Peppermint herb	6 oz

Take 3 capsules twice daily when wife is taking her formula 6 days weekly, for at least 10-12 weeks.

Herbal Combination for Men #2:

Siberian Ginseng, Saw Palmetto, Gotu Kola, Damiana, Sarsaparilla, Horsetail, Ginkgo. Take 3 capsules twice daily.

CHAPTER 3
MISCARRIAGE AND STILLBIRTH

MISCARRIAGE

Miscarriage is the loss of a baby prior to twenty weeks gestation. The majority of miscarriages occur within the first twelve weeks of pregnancy. A study in which the level of pregnancy hormone (beta subunit hCG) was measured in women in the latter end of the luteal phase of their cycles showed physical evidences of pregnancy. This study suggests that many miscarriages occur before a woman is aware she is pregnant, at the time of her regular menstrual cycle.[1]

The main symptoms of miscarriage are vaginal bleeding, spotting, and cramping. Bleeding may be bright red or pink (fresh) or dark brown (old). Two thirds of women who have bleeding unaccompanied by cramps carry their babies to term. If bleeding increases, if cramps or back pain occur at regular intervals, or if a gush of fluid from the vagina occurs, a pregnant woman should consult a qualified health professional immediately.

The cause of a miscarriage may lie with the baby, or with the mother or father. There are seven primary areas that a maternal-fetal medical specialist or reproductive endocrinologist will look to for an explanation of why a woman may have repeated miscarriages:

1. Genetic: Many prospective parents are not comfortable investigating this area, because of the decisions that may be necessitated by the results. Genetic testing is done by taking blood samples from husband and wife to ascertain if either or both of them carry a gene that is causing mutations in their babies. The tests are usually quite expensive, in the

neighborhood of five hundred dollars per individual. If either the husband or wife has family members with genetic abnormalities, or family members who have also experienced a number of miscarriages, this testing may provide missing information. A common pattern in genetically-related problem pregnancies is early-loss miscarriages interspersed with term deliveries, although this is not always so.

2.   Anatomic: An anatomical deviation from the normal interior of a portion of the uterus may cause pregnancy loss. You may wish to investigate this possibility if your mother took DES during her pregnancy—a fairly common drug treatment to prevent miscarriage between 1940 and 1970.

3.   Infectious: Infections with a variety of exotic organisms, as well as more common ones such as the mycoplasmas, can cause pregnancy loss. Most physicians choose to treat this possibility without testing for the organisms, as they can be difficult to culture. The woman is usually treated with doxycycline, taking 100 mg twice daily from day one through to day seven of the cycle in which conception is desired.

4.   Hormonal: A hormonal cause of miscarriage is likely if pregnancy losses are occurring before ten weeks' gestation, particularly from the sixth to the eighth week. Testing for this possible cause of miscarriage takes place during a menstrual cycle through which the basal body temperature is monitored. The woman's progesterone level is measured on the twenty-first day of her cycle. If it is is lower than 15 ng/ml, treatment is usually given in the form of 50-400 mg of natural progesterone, inserted vaginally, until the tenth to twelfth week of pregnancy, beginning on the second evening after the luteal shift signifying ovulation (or the second evening of the color change indicating ovulation in an ovulation-predictor test). If a woman chooses to use the progesterone suppositories, she may want to wean off them over a week's time, rather than abruptly stopping, as theoretically there is a risk of pregnancy loss because of sudden progesterone withdrawal. Doctors do not generally agree that this is a risk factor: they feel that, once the placenta is well established at the tenth week, there is no further need to supplement with progesterone.

5.   Immunologic: Several antibodies can be produced in a woman's body that could increase her risk of miscarriage. These can be identified through blood tests: the anti-coagulant antibody test; prothrombin time test, which checks for blood coagulation disorders; antinuclear antibody tests; and rheumatoid factors, which can indicate rheumatoid diseases that prevent pregnancy or cause pregnancy loss.

6.   Metabolic: A screening for diabetes is normal, as diabetes can cause miscarriages. The thyroid is also usually tested, because low thyroid function levels are associated with increased pregnancy loss. Some physicians prescribe 0.1 mg of synthroid daily, even if the thyroid tests are borderline, or for a woman with previous abnormal thyroid results, just to take care of any possible problems. Other physicians disagree with this "empirical" practice of medicine. Empirical medicine is not based upon clear clinical evidence of need, but rather

on past clinical experience of the therapy being used successfully. I tend to fall into the "empirical" camp on this one. As a woman who has experienced a number of miscarriages, I prefer to think I am doing everything possible to care for my baby in the womb.

7. Environmental: An evaluation of possible toxins in the home or work environment is done to exclude this as a possible cause of recurrent miscarriage.

Since the focus of this book is on natural therapies that may help in certain health conditions, we will address now the healthy aspects of sound nutrition and supplementation that may also be a factor in miscarriage. Normal function of all endocrine glands is important for maintaining a healthy pregnancy; therefore, it is prudent for mothers, and would-be mothers, first of all to provide their bodies with healthful foods.

Lifestyle and dietary recommendations:

1. Bed rest: While there is no definitive evidence that this has any effect on the outcome, many caregivers feel that limiting activity has some physiologic benefit. I feel it certainly has emotional benefit in helping a woman to feel she is doing everything possible to save her baby.
2. No intimate relations: There should be no sexual intercourse until all bleeding has stopped.
3. Nutrition: Continue a high-quality whole foods diet.

Nutritional Supplements:

1. Black haw and crampbark are the two herbs most commonly used by European physicians, Native Americans and modern herbalists to calm the uterus. Prominent naturopaths in Europe even use black haw to counteract the effects of abortifacient drugs.[234] See 5 below for dosage.
2. Red raspberry* has a long history of use in pregnancy for morning sickness, uterine irritability and threatened miscarriage.[5] Standard dosage: 2 capsules 3 times daily. Do not use red raspberry before reading the cautions about Rubus idaeus and prayerfully considering what God allows for your family.
3. False unicorn is prized by herbalists for its adaptogenic effect on the ovaries (it normalizes uterine function), and this has been confirmed by current pharmacology.[6] See 5 below for dosage.
4. Wild yam (Dioscorea villosa) is the basis for commercial birth-control products created by converting Diosgenin (a steroid-like material contained in wild yam species) to progesterone (this conversion from diosgenin to progesterone can only occur in the laboratory; it does not occur within the body when taking wild yam).[7] This herb may benefit those women

who are threatening miscarriage, due to stimulation to the adrenal glands of the body, as well as the antispasmodic effects of the herb.

5. Combination "CarryOn" for Threatened Miscarriage: A combination of black haw, false unicorn, and wild yam (Liquid Light™ or Mother's Choice™). While this combination relaxes the uterine muscle, it does not create a uterus that would prolong an inevitable miscarriage (if the baby had already died). It also helps the body to normalize hormone production. Take 1 teaspoon every 2-3 hours for several hours, then 1/4-1/2 teaspoon once the bleeding and contractions have lessened.

6. Either pasque flower (Anemone pulsatilla) herb or passion flower herb, or both, may be added to the above combination.

7. Other nutrients vital to a healthy pregnancy: essential fatty acids found in natural polyunsaturated (cold-processed) oils such as canola, safflower, soy and flaxseed oils, pumpkin seeds, sunflower seeds, Evening Primrose oil and black currant oil, zinc; magnesium, and vitamin E.

*There has been speculation that the cultivated variety of red raspberry (Rubus idaeus) may be of danger to pregnant women, due to the presence of caffeic acid in the plant that has been shown in one test to inhibit chorionic gonadotropin activity in rats being injected.[8] Other studies clearly show uterine relaxation. The question is whether Rubus idaeus can cause miscarriage in women who are prone to miscarriages. The wild variety of red raspberry (R. stringosus) has been advocated as an alternative to R. idaeus, based on the assumption that it has been safely used throughout history by pregnant women, to add tone to flaccid uteri, and to relax irritable uteri.

I have found no research available on R. stringosus, so it is difficult to validate the claim that it is safer than R. idaeus. It is also not known whether R. stringosus contains caffeic acid, as does R. idaeus. One midwife in Madisonville, Louisiana, DeAnne Domnick, found that a client she was helping through a miscarriage had taken R. idaeus during her pregnancy. She later overheard some students of naturopathy say, "Only idiots use idaeus during pregnancy." Although she was unable to substantiate their crude remark, she feels cautious enough to recommend only R. stringosus to her clients for use during pregnancy.[9]

The Basic CARE Booklets from the Medical Training Institute of America issue a caution about using R. idaeus, as well as recommending R. stringosus, for pregnancy. I was unable to track down the original source of this caution.

From my point of view, I feel it necessary to defend R. idaeus. It is found in almost all herbal combinations, and as a single herb, in liquid or capsule form. It stands to reason that we would see a great increase in miscarriages among women using red raspberry during pregnancy if R. idaeus is indeed a problem. I should also note that those concerned with women using R.

idaeus during pregnancy feel it is only a problem for women prone to miscarriage. A physician working for a nutritional supplement company in Oregon, which has a prenatal formula with R. idaeus in it, said he did not feel that the cultivated variety constituted much of a concern. This was significant coming from him, as he has written several books on herb toxicity.

The problem is that R. stringosis is not widely available. Most herb companies use R. idaeus, and most caregivers educated in herbalism feel comfortable recommending it. Women who have had several miscarriages and want to be very cautious may wish to use R. stringosus, if they can find it. Certainly, though, the cultivated R. idaeus can be taken after the sixteenth week of pregnancy, when hCG levels have stabilized.

STILLBIRTH

When a baby is born dead after twenty weeks' gestation, this is defined as a stillbirth. There are many causes of stillbirths, some particularly due to placental problems, such as placenta abruptio, where the placenta detaches from the uterine wall while the baby is still in utero. Nutritional deficiencies in the mother are evident from the health, or lack thereof, of the placenta. The placenta truly is a window into the environment of the womb. If it does not look healthy, or has anomalies, a woman can purpose to be more diligent about her nutritional intake during her next pregnancy.

There are no nutritional recommendations specific to stillbirth, except the use of zinc supplements as a preventive. I was able to find one study that related vitamin E deficiency to intrauterine growth retardation and prematurity.[10] Apart from these, the best a woman can do is to follow a whole foods diet, and abstain from harmful practices such as alcohol intake, smoking, unnecessary or recreational drug use, and environmental teratagens.

Certainly all stillbirths are not caused by lack of good nutrition. There are many cases that are simply unexplainable.

Where is God in this? Spiritual and emotional, and practical responses

Stillbirth or miscarriage is not just missing carrying a baby to term. It is the loss of life, the life of a child. My own miscarriages have been a mixed bundle, so to speak. My first and my last were the most traumatic. Those in between were not easy, but I did not experience the same amount of grief, perhaps because I knew I was pregnant longer with the first and last, babies we named Sarah and Abel.

My husband and I chose to acknowledge the lives of our children who died in the womb, even those very early miscarriages. We did this in a number of ways:

● Naming our children: For those documented miscarriages, when I knew for certain I was pregnant, we felt it important to give names to those children. Since the miscarriages occurred too early in pregnancy for us to know whether the child was a boy or girl, we prayed, and chose a name based on which we felt the child to be. If we are wrong, that won't affect the eternal scheme of things. This has allowed us to call those children by name in remembrance. It also gives a concrete validation of their lives, which served the purpose for which God created them.

● Family ceremony and burial: We did not do this with all of our miscarriages, but we did with the last ones. A dear friend reminded me to save the baby, or what we could retrieve, which we kept in extreme cold until the ceremony could take place. We used a biodegradable box for the burial, and wrapped the baby in a blanket before allowing our other children to participate. They chose to draw pictures, or to place something special in with the baby. We then had a short service, consisting primarily of affirmation, through prayer, of God's sovereignty, mercy and comfort over, and for, our family. Together, we chose a special stone to mark the grave of our child. Of course, all families will not be able to do this, because of where their home is located.

* Talking about the hopes and dreams we had for that child: With our first miscarriage, Keith and I sat down together to talk about the disappointment we were feeling at the loss of our baby daughter, Sarah. I had already begun buying little baby booties, and clothes that I looked forward to dressing her in; dreaming of how it would feel to hold a sweet little girl in my arms. Keith and I were able to talk of our sadness while at the same time encouraging one another to trust in wisdom of the Lord of All Creation for our lives.

* Let others know our needs: physical, emotional, and spiritual. We knew, particularly this last time, that a woman's body does not realize there is no baby to hold or nurse. The body does react to having been pregnant, and having gone through labor, just as if it had been a term pregnancy. Following a miscarriage or stillbirth, a woman has to take it easy for a week or two, just as if she had her baby with her. We asked our church for help with meals and cleaning for a couple of weeks, as well as letting them share in our grief and encourage us with prayer.

These are some of the steps we took as we dealt with our babies' deaths. You may not feel comfortable with all or even any of the above. However, all parents should know they may grieve as any parents do who have lost a child. The pro-life movement would probably gain more ground were it to acknowledge the lives of children who die within the womb of natural causes, as well as those taken forcibly by the abortionist's hand.

I wish there were an answer we could grasp to explain why we must go through the painful experiences of miscarriage or stillbirth. I was able to take great comfort in Psalm 139, knowing that God formed my babies just as He desired, for His Divine purpose. He numbered each one's days before the baby was even formed. God is good, and His work in me and my family is holy and just. Therefore, as painful as is the death of a baby, God still redeems my baby's life for His good and holy purpose.

Part Four:
Problems With Menses

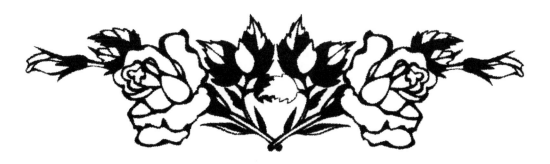

Chapter 1
Acne

Many women experience a problem with acne during early puberty and throughout the teen years. Some continue to have problems with acne throughout their lifetime. The influence of monthly hormonal flux makes oil-secreting glands overactive. There are two types of acne: acne vulgaris, which affects the hair follicles and oil-secreting glands, producing blackheads, whiteheads, and inflammation; and acne conglobata, which causes deep cyst formation with scarring. The most common form is acne vulgaris. The male sex hormone testosterone is the major hormonal factor in acne, causing sebaceous, or sebum-producing, glands to enlarge and produce more sebum. The skin of patients with acne shows increased activity of the enzyme 5-alpha-reductase, which converts testosterone to dihydrotestosterone, a more potent form of the hormone.

Lifestyle and dietary recommendations:

1. Wash your pillowcases in a natural laundry liquid detergent.
2. Switch to a water-based makeup foundation, and other oil-free cosmetics.
3. Wash your face twice daily with a non-soap cleanser, to remove excess oil and sebum. There are cleansing bars available in regular department stores or supermarkets that do not contain soap, and there are certainly natural cleansers that are nourishing and healing to the skin.

4. Follow the whole foods diet. Eliminate sugar, foods containing trans-fatty acids such as milk, milk products, margarine, shortening and synthetically-hydrogenated vegetable oils, fried foods and chocolate. Add anti-acne foods: butternut, sunflower seeds, brazil nuts, pumpkin, soybeans, cashews, pistachios, avocados, breadfruit, black currant, asparagus, chickpea, black beans, lettuce, strawberries, kale.[1]

5. Eat coldwater fish, such as salmon, several times a week, or perhaps add some quality fish oils to your diet.

Nutritional supplement recommendations:

1. A quality vitamin-mineral formula providing daily: zinc 30-45 mg (the daily maximum is 50-75 mg), vitamin A 10,000 IU (a temporary amount of 25,000 to 50,000 IU daily may be used), vitamin E 400 IU, B_6 150 mg in combination with other B vitamins, selenium 200 mcg, and Vitamin B_6 50-100 mg daily. If your multi-formula does not supply all of these nutrients, add single vitamins and minerals to satisfy these requirements.

2. A daily supplement of vitex agnus-castus to help with premenstrual acne. 1-2 capsules each morning, or 40 drops of the liquid extract each morning, taken throughout the menstrual cycle. No drug interactions.

3. Apply Australian tea tree oil topically. A study conducted at the Royal Prince Hospital in New South Wales, Australia, found that a 5% tea tree oil solution demonstrated beneficial effects similar to those of 5% benzoyl peroxide, but with substantially fewer side effects.[2][3] For more serious forms of acne, try up to a 15% tea tree oil solution. Anything of a stronger concentration may irritate the skin. Avoid contact with eyes. No drug interactions.

4. Pantothenic acid supplementation has been shown to cure acne vulgaris completely, if given liberally.[4] May interact with tricyclic antidepressants.

5. A topical extract of hawthorn to be effective in the treatment of acne.[5] May interact with the drug digoxin, generic/trade name Lanoxin.

6. Since allopathic treatment commonly employs antibiotics to treat acne successfully, a natural alternative might be to use the herbs echinacea, 1,000 mg daily, and burdock, 1,000-2,000 mg daily, to stimulate immune activity. Both herbs act on the skin, as well as showing antibacterial actions.

CHAPTER 2
ANEMIA

Anemia is a condition in which the blood does not contain an adequate amount of red blood cells, or hemoglobin—the iron-containing portion of red blood cells. The function of the red blood cell (RBC) is to transport oxygen from the lungs to the tissues of the body, and to exchange it there for carbon dioxide. Symptoms of anemia range from pallor, fatigue, vertigo (dizziness), headache, ringing in the ears, a racing or irregular heartbeat, an inability to breathe easily after physical exertion, to simply feeling as though there is not enough air for even the simple task of walking up a set of stairs. There are many types of anemia; the most common are associated with a deficiency of iron, folic acid, and B_{12}. These are the types we will address.

Iron-deficiency anemia:

A woman with low hemoglobin levels usually experiences symptoms such as fatigue, pale fingernail beds, pale membranes under the eyelids, and pica—the desire to eat ice, corn starch or clay. Some degree of anemia is assumed to be a natural part of pregnancy. Anne Frye, in her book Understanding Diagnostic Tests in the Childbearing Year, states that, because of the physiologic dilution of red blood cells caused by increasing plasma volume, it looks like iron or hemoglobin levels are falling.[1] What actually takes place is that, during the first twenty-eight weeks of pregnancy, a woman's total blood volume expands to meet the needs of her baby, giving the appearance of anemia in blood tests. For women outside of pregnancy, anemia is generally caused by heavy menstrual periods, malnutrition, or genetic predisposition. Sometimes, anemia can be the result of slow internal bleeding from ulcers in the stomach or other areas. For women with heavy periods, the recommendations in Part Three, Chapter 3: Menstrual Dysfunction, in the section dealing with menorrhagia, may be followed to help control the amount of menstrual flow. Women with malnutrition and family predisposition to anemia can control the problem primarily through diet and nutritional supplements.

Megaloblastic anemia:

Megaloblastic anemia is caused by folic acid deficiency or vitamin B_{12} deficiency.

Folic acid deficiency: This type of anemia is most common in those who eat few or no fresh green vegetables. The most noticeable symptom is the "mask of pregnancy"—brown spots on the face—as well as other pigment changes. It may also cause vomiting and loss of appetite. Since folic acid has been found to be instrumental in preventing neural tube defects, supplementation of this nutrient ideally should begin three months before pregnancy.

B_{12} deficiency: B_{12} is a water-soluble vitamin, the only vitamin produced only by bacteria. It is a cobalt-containing substance, so is produced only where there is adequate cobalt available. B_{12} contributes to protein, fat, and carbohydrate metabolism, and is necessary for the normal functioning of the nervous system.

Dietary absorption of B_{12} is highly dependent on the source, and how well an individual body assimilates it. Several factors may contribute to impaired B_{12} absorption:

a) Insufficient hydrochloric acid in the stomach: correct by stimulating acid formation with herbs: peppermint, cayenne, papaya, or bromelain, or supplementing with hydrochloric acid. Adequate salt intake is necessary for acid production.

b) Compromised pancreatic function: correct by balanced calcium supplementation.

c) Pancreas-related malabsorption problem stemming from inhibition of the proteases (protein digesting enzymes): correct with the enzyme trypsin.

d) High heat in cooking, which destroys B_{12}.

e) A diet high in fat, excess mucous-forming foods, and refined foods.

f) Exposure to cigarette smoke, alcohol, birth control pills, nitrous oxide (dental anesthetic gas or auto emissions), mercury amalgam dental fillings, and certain antibiotics (such as Neomycin).

g) Pectin and vitamin C can both destroy B_{12}, while cellulose (dietary fiber) enhances absorption.[2]

h) Food sources that are low in B_{12}: while it has been assumed that people who eat meat have no risk of B_{12} deficiency, research in the past few years has uncovered a decrease in the amount of B_{12} in foods normally rich in B_{12}, such as cheese and liver. This may be due to soils low in cobalt, producing cobalt-deficient plants that stock animals graze on, which in turn produces B_{12}-deficient animals. They can't give what they don't have. Vegetarians also need to ensure they have an adequate B_{12} intake, since plant sources may be cobalt deficient.

Lifestyle and Dietary Recommendations for all three types of anemia:

1. Cook with iron skillets.
2. Follow a whole foods diet.
3. Add the following foods to your diet: prunes, apricots, black cherries, dark, leafy greens (particularly organic dandelion greens), sea vegetables, fermented foods (soy sauce, miso, tamari, etc.), molasses, grapes, almonds, beets, organ meats (absolutely only from certified organic sources). If you eat liver, make certain it is certified organic calf liver, and eat no more than 4 ounces per week.
4. Do not eat the following foods at the same time as you take your iron supplement, as they inhibit iron absorption: bran from whole grains, tea, coffee, caffeinated sodas, calcium-rich antacids, eggs, milk and other dairy products, soy protein, particularly soy milk, and tofu.

Nutritional Supplement Recommendations:

1. Nettle leaf, red raspberry and oat straw infusion: steep an ounce of each herb in 2 quarts of boiled water for at least 4 hours, to make a strong infusion. Drink ½-1 cup several times daily. For those who do not wish to drink an infusion, these herbs may be purchased in capsules, singly or in combination. Take 300-500 mg 2-3 times daily. All of these herbs are high in iron and vitamin C, which aids in the absorption of iron. They are also a good source of chlorophyll. For those who like anise, 1 teaspoon of seeds may be added to the infusion. A 1990 study showed that anise enhances iron absorption.[3] Nettles and oat straw are not associated with any drug interactions. Red raspberry may cause decreased absorption of the following drugs: ephedrine, atropine, theophylline and codeine.
2. Taking a vitamin C and bioflavonoid supplement when taking iron supplements aids absorption.
3. Vitamin E supplementation at 600 IU daily for 30 days may reverse anemia, because of vitamin E's ability to reduce the fragility of red blood cells.[4]
4. Alfalfa leaves, kelp powder and dandelion are high in iron and chlorophyll, as well as a wealth of other minerals. Alfalfa is an excellent source of vitamins A and D, and is a rich source of vitamin K. It has been used in medicine to enhance blood clotting. Dandelion

may interact adversely with the following drugs: thiazide diuretics, spironolactone, loop diuretics, and triamterene.

5. Spirulina and chlorella both contain high amounts of protein and B vitamins, especially folic acid. Spirulina is the best vegetable source of B_{12}. The powder, although not the tastiest thing in the world, is the best way of taking these nutritive foods. Take 2-4 tablespoons of the powder, or 6-12 tablets or capsules, daily.

6. The liquid TincTract™, called Tri-Iron by Tri-Light, contains the herbs yellow dock, dandelion, raspberry, nettles and anise. This combination supplies excellent levels of iron along with herbs added to enhance absorption. Dandelion may interact adversely with the same drugs mentioned in recommendation 4.

7. Yellow dock, alone or in combination with other herbs mentioned above, can be helpful for anemia that is unresponsive to other measures. The dock plant family does contain anthraquinones (chemical constituents that stimulate intestinal peristalsis), just as cascara sagrada does, so one would not want to overdo the dosage. One 450 mg capsule may be taken 2-3 times daily. If diarrhea occurs, reduce the dosage by one capsule.

8. Chlorophyll, in capsule or liquid form, has been used by herbalists to encourage a quick hemoglobin rise, as the molecular structure of chlorophyll is very similar to our hemoglobin. We don't know exactly why this product works so well, but it does. Take 2-3 capsules, or ½-1 cup of the liquid, daily.

9. The multivitamin/mineral supplement should contain adequate iron, folic acid and B_{12} in absorbable forms: iron as citrate, gluconate or fumarate; folic acid as folacin; B_{12} as cobalamin.

10. I have used this herbal combination in capsules throughout my healthy pregnancies to prevent anemia: red beetroot, yellow dock root, red raspberry leaves, chickweed herb, burdock root, nettle herb and mullein leaves. Note the red raspberry drug interactions in recommendation 1.

11. Many midwives have found the supplement called Floridix with iron, or Liquid Herbal Iron, a mix of fruit and herb concentrates, to reverse anemia in the pregnant woman. This could be used by any woman with anemia.

12. Some women will have to try several different therapies to achieve positive results, or even use several at one time. Exercising daily or at least 3 times per week helps increase the oxygen supply to the body, which will help raise hemoglobin levels.

13. For women with extremely low B_{12} levels, one 1000 mcg injection may make all the difference in the world.

CHAPTER 3
MENSTRUAL DYSFUNCTION

AMENORRHEA

Amenorrhea is the term used for lack of menstrual periods. It is called primary amenorrhea in a woman who has never had a menstrual period, and secondary amenorrhea when periods were normal and have stopped. This section will deal with secondary amenorrhea only. If periods are merely irregular—once every two months or so—treatment may not be necessary. If a cycle does not occur for three or more months, the following recommendations may be implemented. These recommendations are based on herbs that supply the necessary building blocks to enable our glands to produce the hormones that regulate menses. The nutritional focus is to support the body's functioning with high-quality proteins and fats.

The most obvious cause of amenorrhea is pregnancy, and a pregnancy test should be performed to rule out pregnancy before a woman begins any of the recommended supplementation. Another cause of amenorrhea that needs no nutritional intervention is postpartum amenorrhea, a normal occurance in breastfeeding mothers. Postpartum amenorrhea may last only six weeks in women who do not breastfeed. However, mothers who breastfeed exclusively—no formula, other foods, water or pacifiers—and who breastfeed at least every two to three hours until the baby begins eating other foods, experience an average of fifteen months without periods (which means no ovulation). Postpartum amenorrhea and natural child spacing are discussed more completely in Part Two, Chapter 1: Well WomanCare.

Lifestyle and Dietary Recommendations:

1. We can become so focused on limiting fats and meats that we deprive our bodies of these necessary foods. A whole foods diet will supply the correct amount of protein and fat without overloading the body.
2. Limit exercise. Long distance runners and ballet dancers, as well as some swimmers, experience amenorrhea due to the amount they exercise. If amenorrhea occurs after beginning a weight-loss regimen, a woman may want to limit exercise to 30 minutes, 3-5 times weekly.
3. If basal body temperature is consistently low, have tests to rule out hypothyroidism as a factor.
4. Emotional stress can be a cause of amenorrhea or irregular cycles. Prayer, relaxation techniques, and discussing matters of concern with your husband and church elders may prove helpful.

Nutritional Supplement Recommendations:

1. Chaste berry, in preliminary investigations, has been shown to adjust the production of female hormones by the presence of several compounds, including a progesterone-like compound[1] [2]. Chaste berry is now believed to have dopaminergic properties: this means it inhibits the secretion of the peptide hormone prolactin, which is produced in large quantities by the pituitary gland[3] in breastfeeding women, and is thought to be responsible for postpartum amenorrhea associated with breastfeeding. Some women who are not breastfeeding have high levels of prolactin, which cause the normal menstrual cycle to cease. Dosage: at least 20 mg standardized tablets or capsules daily.
2. Mugwort has been used in many different countries, including the United States, to assist and promote menstruation. Test-tube experiments confirm that it does contract uterine tissue, but human studies are lacking. [4] Dosage: 2 capsules daily.
3. In my own counseling on herb use, I have found a product, Fem-a-Gen by Rainbow Light, to regulate the menses, even in cases where women were previously using strong medications to bring on their menstrual cycles. Dosage on the bottle may be followed.
4. Dong quai has a tonic effect on the uterus, making it useful for many menstrual disorders, including amenorrhea. Dosage: 2-3 capsules daily.
5. One study has shown that 2 g per day of acetyl-L-carnitine for 6 months had a positive impact on menstruation.[5]

DYSMENORRHEA

Dysmenorrhea is the medical term used to describe painful menstrual periods, with cramps in the lower abdominal area. While most women experience some discomfort during menstruation, those who must restrict normal activities due to cramping are diagnosed as having dysmenorrhea. Approximately fifty percent of women of childbearing age experience dysmenorrhea. Out of these, one in five are incapacitated from one to three days each month because of pain.[6] Herbs have been found to be of great benefit to women who seek relief from monthly menstrual pain. The most important factor in herbal care of this condition—and many other conditions as well—is beginning the nutritional supplement of your choice at the first hint of a cramp. Women who have very regular cycles may want to begin their herbal therapy a day or two prior to when their menstrual flow will begin.

Lifestyle and Dietary Recommendations:

1. Foods containing arachidonic acid should be limited or avoided during the week prior to and during menstruation. Arachidonic acid is converted in the body to the PGE prostaglandin, which causes the uterine muscles to contract. Animal foods are the primary—in fact, almost the only—source of arachidonic acid. (Humans produce arachidonic acid, but I hope there is no chance of you eating your neighbor!)
2. Limit dairy products. They contain arachidonic acid and calcium, which cause muscles to contract.
3. Increase foods containing magnesium: whole grains, beans, nuts. Magnesium causes muscles to relax.
4. A warm lavender, chamomile or passion flower bath may be helpful, to aid relaxation.
5. A hot water bottle, warm towels, and warm clothing are always preferable to cold items, which cause all tissues to contract. I have found that having my husband wet a towel and microwave it until it is very warm (just not hot enough to burn me) and placing it on my abdomen or back can provide instant relief from the worst of cramping.

Nutritional Supplement Recommendations:

1. Evening Primrose oil capsules are an excellent choice for women with dysmenorrhea. This oil has a high gamma-linolenic acid (GLA) content, which converts to the "good" prostaglandins—those that cause the uterine muscles to relax. Take 1-2 capsules of 500 mg, 3 times daily.

2. Red raspberry leaf tea or capsules have long been used to reduce cramping during menstrual cycles. Take 2-6 capsules daily. Red raspberry may decrease absorption of the following drugs: ephedrine, theophylline, atropine and codeine.

3. Pain-relieving herbs such as white willow bark and meadowsweet may be of benefit, as they help lower the pain-causing prostaglandins.

4. Valerian root and cramp bark are two valuable herbs scientifically documented to relax smooth muscle. Take 1-2 capsules of each, every 2-3 hours while experiencing cramps. Frontier Herbs has a formula that features valerian root and cramp bark.

5. CrampEase by TriLight Herbs works well for cramps and after-birth pains. The herbs contained in this combination are crampbark or black haw, valerian, skullcap, hops, catnip, and chamomile. Take ½-1 teaspoon every 2-3 hours during a painful cycle.

6. Female Formula by TriLight Herbs is also helpful for relieving painful menstruation.

7. FemCare by Enzymatic Therapy was specifically formulated for use during menstruation to relieve pain.

8. Another product providing significant relief from the cramping is Fem-a-Gen by Rainbow Light. I have found taking 2-3 capsules at the onset of menstrual pain brings maximum relief.

9. For the nausea and vomiting that sometimes accompany severe menstrual cramping, ginger root may help, at a dosage of 2-3 capsules every 2-3 hours. Ginger has the added benefit of being anti-inflammatory, cutting down on the cramp-promoting prostaglandins, as well as helping to reduce intestinal and uterine cramping. Although there have been no reports of adverse interactions with drugs that are anti-coagulants (blood thinners), you may want to discuss the use of ginger with your physician before taking it with heparin, warfarin, or ticlopidine.

MENORRHAGIA

Menorrhagia refers to heavy blood loss during menstrual periods. It can sometimes be debilitating, as a woman is loathe to keep up with normal activities when she is constantly concerned about bleeding through to her clothes. Excessively prolonged menstrual flow—lasting more than six or seven days—is now called "hypermenorrhea."

Menorrhagia can be due to a variety of factors: endometriosis, uterine fibroids, low thyroid function, nutrient deficiencies, post-birth control pill hormone changes, or reproductive tract tumors or cysts. Menorrhagia may also be simply a few days of extremely heavy bleeding. If left unchecked, heavy bleeding can lead to anemia. Nutritional changes and an herbal treatment protocol should be coupled with medical testing to rule out a more serious health condition, if the heavy bleeding or irregular periods of bleeding last for more than three months.

Any vaginal blood flow that causes a woman to soak through a maxipad in thirty minutes or less is cause for an immediate trip to the emergency room. Bleeding between normal periods is termed "metrorrhagia" and should be evaluated by a medical professional.

Lifestyle and Dietary Recommendations:

1. Eat a large salad of dark, green leafy vegetables every day, to supply vitamin K, iron, folic acid, vitamin A, and chlorophyll, which are all needed in greater amounts when bleeding has occurred.
2. Include sea vegetables in the diet, such as kelp, dulse, spirulina, etc., which provide nutrients for the endocrine (glandular) system.
3. Commit to the whole foods diet for at least 6 months, to allow time for the body to recuperate and adjust to better quality foods.
4. Have your thyroid function checked, and treat with natural thyroid glandular supplements or synthetic thyroid hormones as necessary to control the condition.

Nutritional Supplement Recommendations:

1. There are several formulas that nourish the female endocrine system. A formula containing the following herbs has proven beneficial for many women: Chaste berry (Vitex agnus castus), wild yam, dong quai, licorice, ginger, Blue Cohosh (may elevate blood pressure) or Black Cohosh, as well as liver-supportive herbs such as dandelion, milk thistle, burdock and/or yellow dock. Cautions: dong quai can be taken from ovulation to the onset of menstruation, but should be discontinued after menstruation begins if it leads to heavy bleeding. Definitely avoid dong quai during menstruation if you have fibroids. This herb

may also aggravate bloating or diarrhea, and should not be taken with thrombolytic or blood-thinning medications. Dong quai should not be taken with anti-coagulant drugs such as heparin, warfarin and ticlopidine. Licorice may decrease the clearance of prednisone, thus possibly increasing the risk of prednisone-related side effects, and may increase the side effects of potassium-depleting diuretics, including thiazide and loop diuretics (Deglycyrrhizinated licorice [DGL] may be used safely with all diuretics). Excessive use of licorice may cause the body to lose potassium, which could possibly increase the risk of digoxin toxicity.

2. Several herbs have traditionally been used to halt uterine bleeding. The following herbs have demonstrated the ability to curb bleeding: shepherd's purse, yarrow, cayenne pepper (may stimulate bleeding later if not used in combination with a styptic herb such as shepherd's purse), and bayberry. These herbs are contained in the HemHalt™ by TriLight Herbs.

3. Chlorophyll has long been used for bleeding because of its similar molecular structure to human blood. Whether this is why chlorophyll works well in slowing down bleeding or rebuilding blood supply after bleeding episodes is unknown. Midwives have long used it in cases of hemorrhage. Take 2-3 capsules daily, or ½-1 cup of liquid daily.

4. A high-quality vitamin supplement is a must for women with excessive bleeding. The brands I like best are NF Women's Formula by NF Formulas, and Opti-Natal by Eclectic Institute. There are many good multivitamins on the market. The supplement you choose must have an adequate amount of vitamin A, as vitamin A deficiency has been shown to be a causative factor in menorrhagia.[7]

CHAPTER 4
MIGRAINES

An ache in the head, or headache, occurs when pain arises from the outer lining of the brain and scalp and its blood vessels and muscles. There are essentially two types of headaches: migraine, or vascular headache, and tension headache, which is characterized by a steady, constant, dull pain that starts at the back of the head or forehead and spreads over the entire head, with a sense of pressure being applied to the skull.

Migraine headaches:
* may be triggered by hormonal changes (possibly progesterone excess prior to the onset of menstrual flow), family history, stressful situations or even foods;
* are characterized by "classic" migraine symptoms: throbbing, pounding, sharp pain, usually starting and staying on one side of the head, though it is possible for the pain to spread to both sides; localized pain behind one eye;
* are preceded sometimes, and in some women, by warning signs: vision changes such as halos around objects or people, a tingling sensation, altered perceptions, and strange moods;
* are usually accompanied by some form of abdominal discomfort: gas spasms, nausea and/or vomiting.

Interestingly, migraines typically occur in the morning on weekends and holidays, peak within four to twenty-four hours, and fade gradually. Some migraines begin with an increase in serotonin, a hormone produced in the brain and from blood platelets, which causes constriction of the blood vessels and triggers platelets to release more serotonin, elevating the problem. You can find out if this scenario fits you by taking in some form of caffeine at the onset of your migraine: if it helps, then the herb periwinkle should help you to control your migraines.

Lifestyle and Dietary Recommendations:

1. Allergy is the major cause of migraines.[1] The same allergens can cause tension headaches as well. Common allergens are: milk, wheat, chocolate, food additives, MSG, artificial sweeteners like aspartame, tomatoes and fish.
2. Chocolate, cheese, beer, wine and aspartame may cause migraines, because they contain vasoactive amines that cause blood vessels to expand. Many migraine sufferers are found to have low levels of the platelet enzyme that normally breaks down dietary amines. Tyramine is present in these foods, which is an amino acid found to increase the release of serotonin.

Nutritional Supplement Recommendations:

1. Magnesium deficiency is known to set the stage for migraines and tension headaches.[2] One function of magnesium is to maintain tone of blood vessels. Women need 350-500 mg of magnesium aspartate or citrate daily.
2. Feverfew, while not to be used during pregnancy because of its emmenagogue properties (it promotes menstruation and is considered an abortifacient), has been used for centuries for headaches. Modern research continues to confirm its historical use. A 1988 survey found 70% of 270 migraine sufferers who ate feverfew daily for prolonged periods claimed that the herb decreased the frequency and/or intensity of the attacks. This prompted clinical trials at the London Migraine Clinic, a double-blind study in which patients reported they were helped by feverfew. Those receiving a placebo had a significantly increased frequency and severity of their headaches, nausea and vomiting during the six months of study. Two patients in the placebo group who had been in complete remission during self-treatment with feverfew said they had developed recurrence of incapacitating migraines, and had to withdraw from the study. Self-treatment renewed remission in both patients.[3] A second double-blind study at the University of Nottingham showed feverfew to be effective in reducing the number and severity of migraine attacks.[4] Feverfew works by inhibiting the release of blood vessel-dilating substances from platelets, inhibiting production of inflammatory substances, and re-establishing blood vessel tone.[5] Parthenolide is thought to be the active ingredient. To achieve the same results as those in the studies, you need to take a capsule containing at least 0.2% of parthenolide per 25 mg of freeze-dried pulverized leaves twice daily, or 82 mg dried powdered leaves once daily. A higher dose of 1-2 g is needed during an acute attack. No side effects have been reported as long as the leaves are

not chewed. This may result in small ulcerations in the mouth, and swelling of the lips and tongue, in 10% of users.

3. Nitrites may cause headaches, according to neurologists William P. Henderson and Neil H. Raskin, of the University of California at San Francisco. If a woman is prone to headaches, she needs to watch out for hot dogs, bacon, salami, ham and other meats cured with sodium nitrite or nitrate.[6] These foods are not the best for a pregnant woman to choose anyway, since they can be contaminated with campylobacter bacteria, which can cause miscarriage or stillbirth.

4. Caffeine has been referred to as the nation's Number One headache instigator, says Dr. David W. Buchholz, director of the Neurological Consultation Clinic at Johns Hopkins University Hospital. Although some tests have shown small amounts of caffeine to be able to relieve headaches by temporarily constricting dilated and swollen blood vessels, the vessels swell up and dilate in a rebound action, worsening the headache. The other problem with caffeine is that it is addictive, and most people experience caffeine withdrawal headaches as well as fatigue, mild depression, nausea and vomiting. Withdrawal symptoms usually start 12-24 hours after ceasing caffeine consumption, and are usually over in a week.[7] To get off caffeine without going through severe withdrawal, mix regular and decaffeinated coffee over a week's period, increasing the amount of decaf each day until it is all decaf. Use the same strategy in eliminating tea and sodas. It is a good idea to wean off the decaf versions of these drinks after you overcome the caffeine hurdle, as the decaf versions have their own health risks.

5. Ginger acts much like aspirin, in that it blocks prostaglandin synthesis, which leads to a reduction in inflammation and pain, according to Dr. Drishna C. Srivastava at Odense University in Denmark. It is safe for both adults and children, with no side effects reported. The recommended amount is 1-2 capsules of 500-600 mg each, taken with water up to four times daily as needed.[8] In China, birth practitioners caution against using too much ginger (20-28 grams = 20,000-28,000 mg) in the early portion of pregnancy, due to its stimulant properties.[9] I could find no scientific documentation of any abortifacient qualities to this herb in the quantities recommended above. Scientific research on ginger does include studies of its use by pregnant women, particularly those with hyperemesis gravidarum— excessive vomiting during pregnancy.

6. Omega-3 fish oils may be a migraine headache preventive. This does not mean you can reach for it as a headache is coming on. To be helpful, the supplement needs to be taken over the long term in those who are prone to migraine attacks.[10]

CHAPTER 5
ANXIETY AND DEPRESSION

Anxiety and depression are common problems among women in our society. Our day-to-day responsibilities can seem overwhelming. All too often we lack the spiritual instruction that could help us to be content in all our circumstances, even as the apostle Paul was amidst great adversity as he preached the gospel throughout the world. Too much preaching tells us we can expect life to be kind as long as we are believers. This flies in the face of the Word of God, where we are specifically and repeatedly told to expect people to revile us because we serve Christ and not the world. We can expect adversities to be a regular occurrence in our lives because we serve Christ and not the world.

The refining process God uses to produce holiness in our lives is not an easy one. Gold has to go through fire in order to be refined—God's Word uses that very analogy to describe our own refining. I have gone through some fires already that threatened to overwhelm me, and I am quite certain more will come. Since I am commanded to be thankful in all things, in all circumstances, I must learn to welcome these adversities. That does not mean having some false sense of happiness when I am going through what may feel like "hell on earth." It does mean I have to be content to walk through it, with Christ by my side, upholding me through each step.

Paul's attitude as he spoke to the Philippians concerning his own adversity was: To live is Christ and to die is gain (Philippians 1:21). That is the attitude we must strive for as we face each new day with its new challenges to our faith. Each day that I live, I live to represent Christ in this world, and if I am to die, then to be with the Savior is only great gain.

Now, this is not to say that all anxiety and depression comes directly from spiritual issues, although I believe the majority does. The physical causes of depression can range from:

● lack of good nutrition: it is difficult to feel good when you don't have the oomph to feel much of anything except the need to lie down;

● PMS: hormonal flux can generate some temporary feelings of anxiety and depression;

● postpartum hormonal changes can produce the temporary state known as "postpartum blues";

● menopause: the body's adjustments to lesser hormonal stimulation can be a major cause of temporary anxiety and depression.

You will notice that I used "temporary" several times when referring to physical causes. This is because I believe that, should anxiety levels continue or increase, or depression lengthen significantly, a base spiritual cause needs to be investigated. I highly recommend the books on this subject by counselor Dr. Jay Adams.

New treatment for anxiety and depression is emerging in herbal medicine as more research is accomplished that confirms the validity of botanical medicine for the treatment of these disorders.

Nutritional Supplement Recommendations:

1. Kava root (Piper methysticum) contains kavalactones, substances that exhibit sedative, analgesic, anticonvulsant and muscle-relaxant effects in laboratory animals. Clinical studies confirm the benefit of using kava extracts for anxiety. Kava does not have the negative effect of decreasing cognitive function as do many antidepressants. Actually, kava improves mental function. Standardized extracts are best so that the amount of kavalactones is measured accurately. To achieve the desired anxiolytic effects, 45-70 mg of kavalactones 3 times daily are needed. For sedative effects, the same daily quantity may be taken all at once, 1 hour before bedtime. Higher dosages are not recommended, as side effects may be noted over a prolonged period. Although kava has been reported to cause problems when mixed with benzodiazepines, this has not been proven. Kava works on the limbic system, a part of the brain involved in regulating mood and wakefulness, which is not the way benzodiazepines function in the body. In the one reported incidence of a man taking benzodiazepines and kava, who arrived at a hospital lethargic and disoriented, it was found that his problem was due more to another drug he was taking, Tagamet, which can alter the metabolic effects of other drugs, and possibly that of herbs.

2. St. John's wort, which contains hypericin and pseudohypericin, may be used as a mild to moderate antidepressant. St. John's wort inhibits both A and B monoamine oxidases (MAO). As a result of this inhibition, there is an increase in the level of nerve impulse transmitters

within the brain that maintain normal mood and emotional stability. St. John's wort is virtually free of side effects at the standard dosage of 300 mg three times daily. St. John's wort may interact with MAO inhibitor antidepressants, as well as SSRI and tricylcic antidepressants.

3. Valerian has been widely used in herbal medicine as a sedative. Valerian both improves sleep quality and relieves insomnia. As a mild sedative, valerian extract (0.8% valeric acid) can be taken 30-45 minutes before bedtime, at a dosage of 150-300 mg. The best supplements are water-soluble extracts standardized for valeric acid content.

CHAPTER 6
PREMENSTRUAL SYNDROME

Premenstrual syndrome (PMS) seems to be the most commonly discussed malady of menstruating women in our culture. Modern feminist thought seeks to rob us of the joy of womanhood and, so, has turned natural hormone fluctuations in many women into a disease-state or syndrome. Hormone levels do naturally fluctuate each month, bringing with those fluctuations naturally occurring bodily changes: water retention, breast swelling, constipation, emotional high and lows, and fatigue. When these mild changes occur during the second half of the cycle, after ovulation, they are a result of the increase in the hormone progesterone, which helps prepare a woman's uterus for accepting the implantation of a baby. Progesterone produced the effects mentioned above—just ask any pregnant woman who has an adequate supply of progesterone.

I am not saying that premenstrual syndrome is a myth all in a woman's head. What I want to do is point out the difference between natural hormonal fluctuations, and the body changes we can expect to occur with them, and the problem of excess estrogen syndrome, which is what premenstrual syndrome should really be called. We should be able to differentiate between women who have this syndrome and those who are simply experiencing the physiological changes associated with God's perfect design of our bodies.

From this point, we will assume that the disease we call premenstrual syndrome is actually more a problem of excess estrogen levels, which are associated with low adrenal function, and decreased liver and gastrointestinal function.

Current understanding of PMS:

* PMS sufferers have demonstrated a higher sensitivity to and/or higher levels of prolactin—the predominant hormone in breastfeeding women;

* an excess of dietary saturated fats, alcohol and stress all disrupt the pathway of the prostaglandin PGE1, a "good" prostaglandin that counteracts the effects of prolactin, and reduces the dysmenorrheic (menstrual and premenstrual cramping) properties of the series 2 prostaglandins;

* excess estrogen enhances the aldosterone system (renin, angiostensin), causing fluid and salt retention;

* caffeine and other methylxanthines, such as chocolate, inhibit enzymes, raise kinin and histamine levels, and lower vitamin B$_1$ levels, which results in estradiol buildup;

* the liver is responsible for detoxifying the bloodstream of substances such as excess estrogen. When liver function is decreased, estrogen levels rise.

* slow bowel transit time leads to higher levels of estrodiol (estrogen) circulating in the blood, because it is reabsorbed through the intestinal tract and sent back to the liver, where it must be broken down again;

* excess weight reduces the clearance of estrogen, since fat cells release estrogen into the bloodstream;

* thyroid hormone is an estrogen antagonist; therefore, women with low-thyroid hormones have increased estrogen levels.

What becomes obvious is that we must lower excess prolactin and estrogen levels in order to alleviate the symptoms of PMS. How we accomplish these lowered levels is important. Many supplement companies tell us the key is wild yam creme. Other "Dead Doctors" tapes tell us calcium is the key to cure. Nutritionists tout a whole foods, basically vegetarian, diet as the key. Dr. Guy Abraham, the leading researcher into PMS in the United States, assures us through his studies of the effectiveness of a multivitamin supplement as the key. Are we going to spend time trying to use just one of these to see if the key fits the lock, or will we use the master key to open the door?

The master key to alleviating PMS, as I have defined it, is the same as the counsel I give clients for various concerns. A multi-disciplinary approach is needed to achieve total health. This includes: understanding the spiritual aspects of the problem, adjusting the diet to meet the needs of the current health concern, supplementing the diet with nutrients known to alter the course of the disease, and getting adequate physical exercise to facilitate the program. The multi-disciplinary approach to PMS, or excess estrogen syndrome, ensures that we do not leave out a vital part of the health program, or think of one specific "potion" as the cure.

Spiritual Aspects of PMS

My greatest area of concern, when listening to women discuss their PMS symptoms, is the lack of knowledge of the way we are created, by our perfect and all-wise Creator. In order to prepare for, and sustain, pregnancy, which is a blessing bestowed on us, at God's discretion, during our childbearing years—years in which PMS is known to occur!—our bodies must experience a monthly rise in estrogen levels, as they prepare the egg for release and fertilization. These levels peak at ovulation, beginning to decrease as progesterone levels rise to prepare the endometrium—the lining of the uterus—for implantation of a baby.

Mild symptoms that we generally associate with PMS may actually be a sign that our bodies are functioning properly, with adequately rising progesterone levels. Severe symptoms, which interfere with our daily life, may signify an imbalance in our natural hormone levels. These can, and should, be treated with the natural therapies listed below.

Symptoms of PMS

Premenstrual syndrome is a complex of symptoms, which include: headache, breast swelling and tenderness, abdominal bloating, peripheral edema, fatigue, irritability, tension and depression. Other common symptoms are increased thirst and appetite, constipation and acne. PMS symptoms generally begin after ovulation, and linger until menstrual bleeding begins. In severe cases, symptoms may last virtually all month. While the medical community generally maintains this is a syndrome with no cause, leading researchers into PMS name nutritional deficiencies and imbalances as the cause.

The Work of Dr. Guy Abraham

Dr. Abraham has divided PMS sufferers into four categories under the overall label of Premenstrual Tension:
- PMT-A (for anxiety): characterized by nervous tension, mood swings, irritability and anxiety;
- PMT-H (for hyperhydration): characterized by symptoms such as weight gain, swelling of the extremities, breast tenderness, and abdominal bloating;
- PMT-C (for carbohydrate craving): characterized by headaches, craving for sweets, increased appetite, heart pounding, fatigue, and dizziness or faintness;
- PMT-D (for depression): which involves depression, forgetfulness, crying, confusion and insomnia.[1]

Dr. Abraham found that the dietary intake of nutrients in women with premenstrual symptoms is often less than in healthy women with no premenstrual symptoms.

Lifestyle and dietary recommendations:

1. Limit consumption of refined sugar, salt, red meat and alcohol.
2. Eat fish, poultry, whole grains and legumes as major sources of protein, and rely less on red meat and dairy products. Animal products provide a body source for arachadonic acid, which increases pain-causing prostaglandins in our body; they should be limited during the times of the month when PMS is a problem. This primarily vegetarian diet is not necessary for everyone, but may be best for women who experience severe premenstrual symptoms. Other women, with less severe symptoms, may simply want to limit their intake of animal products for 10 days prior to the onset of menstruation.
3. Reduce or eliminate smoking.
4. Bitter vegetables, such as dark green leafy vegetables, help the liver to function in a more efficient manner, leading to greater clearance of estrogen from the system.
5. Consume only minimal quantities of coffee, tea, chocolate and cola-based drinks.
6. Reduce intake of fats, avoiding particularly animal fats, fried foods and hydrogenated margarines.
7. Increase intake of fiber in the form of complex carbohydrates such as green and leafy vegetables, legumes and fruits. Fiber causes excess estrogen to be excreted from the body through normal, regular bowel movements. Without adequate fiber intake, excess estrogen can be reabsorbed into the bloodstream, increasing estrogen levels.
8. Reduce weight, if you are obese, by avoiding refined carbohydrates, reducing animal fat intake, and increasing fiber intake.
9. If you have sugar or other food cravings, try eating high-quality protein snacks, such as nuts, seeds, peas, beans, and lentils, and animal protein in the form of fish, eggs or poultry.
10. Exercise outdoors regularly.
11. Reduce stress.
12. Avoid making major decisions when during the PMS time of your cycles.

Nutritional supplement recommendations:

1. A high-quality multivitamin such as Opti-Gyn by Eclectic Institute: Opti-Gyn has proven scientific value in treating PMS.
2. Evening Primrose oil: 4-8 capsules of 500 mg each per day, beginning 2 weeks before the start of menstruation.
3. Vitamin E: 300-500 IU daily, especially for breast swelling and tenderness.

4. Magnesium: 200-300 mg of magnesium aspartate or citrate every day of the month, combined with the above multivitamin.

5. Fem-a-Gen by Rainbow Light: has also been successfully used to regulate and balance the female hormones.

6. Chaste berry (Vitex agnus-castus): balances the hormones and reduces prolactin levels. Vitex may be taken in standardized form at a dosage of 1 capsule or 40 drops each morning for several months for maximum effectiveness. In its crude form, as a powdered herb, 2-3 capsules each morning may be needed to obtain the necessary potency.

7. Dong quai: while it has estrogenic properties, it serves more medicinally as an adaptogen, helping to regulate the female hormones rather than acting in the body as a certain hormone. Take 500 mg daily. Do not combine dong quai with anticoagulant medications such as warfarin, heparin and ticlopidine. Discontinue use if heavy bleeding occurs.

8. Feverfew: for migraines, if they are a part of your PMS symptoms. This herb should be taken daily throughout the month in order for it to decrease migraine occurrence. Feverfew should not be taken during pregnancy, due to its abortifacient effect.

Is Natural Progesterone the Answer?

No—according to a study by Sampson in 1979. Instead of concentrating on administering progesterone to try to balance the excess estrogen levels, we should focus our strategy on reducing excess estrogen, specifically estradiol. This makes supplementation with natural progesterone creme, developed from wild yam, not the best choice for a PMS supplementation program. If the creme is used as part of a complete program to decrease excess estrogen through diet, lifestyle and herbs, and increase progesterone, it should only be used after ovulation during the cycle when it is needed. As with any other herb product, it should only be used medicinally when it is needed, not on a daily, long-term basis.

CHOOSING THE BEST PMS MULTI-VITAMIN AND MINERAL SUPPLEMENT:

The information here, while highly technical, is given in order to help you make wise choices at your health food store, through knowing how and why particular supplements work. Your supplement should contain all of the following nutrients:

B-VITAMINS, PARTICULARLY B$_6$: Adams and Abraham have shown that these significantly improve PMS symptoms. B$_6$ is a cofactor for essential fatty acid (EFA) metabolism. It is also important in dopamine formation (dopamine suppresses prolactin, a hormone often elevated in those with PMS) and serotonin production (serotonin helps stabilize mood swings). B$_6$ also acts as a diuretic, reducing hyperpermeability of cell membranes, which decreases interstitial fluid shifts. Elevated estrogen level results in decreased B$_6$ reserves, because estrogen releases hepatic (liver) enzymes, which compete for B$_6$. Therefore, B$_6$ essentially results in improved hepatic clearance of estrogen.

CALCIUM: Blood levels drop in the 14 days prior to menses; therefore, calcium supplementation may help to relieve the insomnia, cramps and headache symptoms of PMS.

CHROMIUM AND MANGANESE: Supplementation with these minerals is important in cases of PMS that are accompanied by marked hyperinsulinism (excessive release of insulin) and resultant hypoglycemia.

ESSENTIAL FATTY ACIDS: The crucial role of EFAs (essential fatty acids) and GLAs (gamma linoleic acids) in the treatment of PMS was outlined by Horrobin in the Journal of Reproductive Medicine, Vol. 28, 1983. With the elevated prolactin levels and low PGE levels in the blood of PMS sufferers, dietary linoleic acid and GLA are required for conversion to PGE 1, which counteracts the effects of prolactin and reduces the dysmenorrheic properties of the series 2 prostaglandins. Conversion of GLA to PGE 1 is accomplished in the body through a biochemical pathway that requires the following cofactors at different steps: B$_6$, magnesium, vitamin C, niacin, and zinc. Sources of GLA include black currant oil and evening primrose oil. While borage oil contains GLA, it also contains pyrillizodine alkaloids, which can be toxic to the liver if used in large quantities over a long period of time, which could be necessary to treat PMS.

LIVER-SUPPORTIVE HERBS: Strengthening and cleansing the liver to aid estrogen reduction may be accomplished through lipotropic factors such as choline, methionine and inositol, as well as the botanicals oregon grape (berberis), celandine (chelidonium), milk thistle (silybum) and dandelion (taraxacum), which improve hepatic circulation, improve digestion and excretion, decrease hepatic congestion and torpor, promote bile formation, promote cholagogue activity, and aid weight loss.

MAGNESIUM: The American Journal of Clinical Nutrition, 1964, reports that magnesium deficiency leads to water retention, causes hyperirritability of muscles, increased urination, and erratic emotional states. In treatment of PMS, the suggested calcium to magnesium ratio is 1:1; 600 mg per day has been found to significantly reduce PMS symptoms.

MILD HERBAL LAXATIVES: Bulk-forming laxatives, such as psyllium, apple pectin or slippery elm, help decrease bowel transit time, which in turn reduces estradiol levels in the bloodstream.

VITAMIN C: Vital for every aspect of our health, vitamin C enhances the activity of enzyme pathways and strengthens cell wall integrity (decreasing abnormal permeability). Bioflavonoids have antihistamine activity, and inhibit estrogen by competing for receptor sites.

VITAMIN D, FOLATE (FOLIC ACID) AND PABA: The supplement you choose should have low levels of these nutrients. In order for the body to properly utilize calcium, one cannot have excessive levels of vitamin D; therefore, it's important not to exceed recommended daily allowances for vitamin D. Folic acid potentiates the action of estrogen, thus intensifying PMS symptoms. PABA should be low because it has anti-thyroid properties (the thyroid provides integral estrogen antagonists).

VITAMIN E AND SELENIUM: Abrahms (1965) found that 400 IU of vitamin E daily prevents oxidation of EFAs, adrenal and sex hormones.

ZINC: Deficiency is common, and causes irritability, depression and skin changes. Copper is needed to balance zinc. Betaine hydrochloride (HCl) increases absorption of zinc. Potassium acts as a diuretic and aids sodium balance (high sodium is associated with PMS). Iron prevents the anemia that is often seen in PMS.

Part Five:
Abnormal Cell Growth

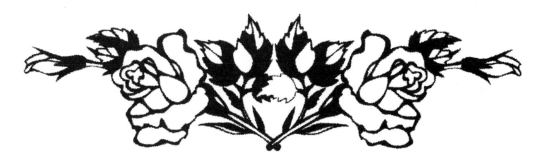

CHAPTER 1
FIBROID TUMORS

Uterine fibroids are benign tumor growths that are generally solid. They can grow in the outer layer of the uterus or the inner portion. Most small fibroids cause no symptoms in a woman, while larger ones can be quite problematic for pregnancy or increasing menstrual bleeding and pain. Uterine fibroids are estrogen dependent, so we know that fertility treatments with estrogenic drugs, oral contraceptives and pregnancy will likely result in increased growth of the fibroid(s). Part of our natural therapy is centered around naturally lowering any excess estrogen levels as well as controlling the pain and excessive menstrual bleeding that may occur.

Fibroid Risk Factors

* Never being pregnant
* Obesity
* Alcohol use
* High-fat diet
* Sedentary lifestyle
* Use of oral contraceptives (birth control pills)
* Other estrogen drugs
* Vitamin B deficiency

Who Gets Fibroids?

The woman who typically gets fibroids is usually between thirty-five and forty-five years of age, who may even have had a family history of fibroid tumors. Fibroids occur in twenty-five percent of white women and fifty percent of black women. Interestingly, black women living in Africa rarely develop fibroids. If a woman has one fibroid tumor, she is eighty-five percent likely to develop more.

Problems They Cause

These growths can become quite large; the largest on record tipped the scales at one hundred and forty pounds. Obviously, carrying around any added weight in an area that is not designed to carry that weight continuously can be a problem, even adding back problems to the array of trouble these tumors can have on a woman's life. Large fibroids can crowd the organs surrounding the uterus, such as the bladder, bowel, kidneys or blood vessels. A woman can even experience a pinched sciatic nerve due to compression by a fibroid.

The most significant problem is heavy menstrual bleeding, with possible severe cramps. The heavy bleeding can lead to anemia, causing pallor and fatigue. Another problem may be miscarriages in a woman with fibroids that grow within the uterus. This is uncommon but should be investigated in a woman with heavy, painful periods who has repeated miscarriages. Very large fibroids may also prevent a vaginal birth, if the fibroid is near the cervix, obstructing the baby's pathway.

Standard Treatment

The first rule of thumb is to rule out uterine cancer. This process usually begins with a pelvic exam, then diagnostic ultrasound. Ultrasonography cannot rule out cancer, but an experienced sonographer can at least give a report on the size and location of the mass and give some idea as to whether further investigation should be done. Hysteroscopy, a diagnostic test where a lighted scope is inserted into the uterus through the cervix so that a doctor may view the interior of the cervix, is done. Other doctors may choose to perform a dilation and curettage (D&C), in which the cervix is dilated and the physician lightly scrapes the uterus to check for tissue changes. More often than not, a woman with suspected fibroids is reexamined every few months for changes in size of the tumor.

In the past, hysterectomy was the only treatment of choice for uterine fibroids. Things have been changing as women are becoming more vocal about hanging on to their internal organs, that many physicians used to think we just didn't need. Even now, fifty percent of hysterectomies are performed due to uterine fibroids. This may be a necessity if heavy menstrual bleeding cannot be controlled through any other method; however, the decision needs to be weighed carefully due to the abrupt surgical menopause that will occur post-surgery, as well as the implications of hormonal replacement therapy on what may be a very young woman.

Some physicians will use laparoscopic surgery to remove only the fibroids and not the entire uterus. Laparoscopy only requires a small incision at the "belly button" and one directly above the pubic bone. Gas is passed into the abdominal cavity to allow the surgeon to insert a camera through one of the incisions and instruments through another to see what he is doing and to actually perform any necessary surgical procedures. This surgery, although still a surgery and significant, may be a better choice than hysterectomy for most women.

Yet another treatment is the use of an anti-estrogenic drug, gonadorelin, to reduce the size of the fibroids. Several studies show that the size of the tumors may be reduced by up to ninety percent in three or four months with the drug. The drug does have some serious drawbacks in that, with any decrease in estrogen levels, it can cause an increased risk for a woman of loss of bone mass, greater susceptibility to heart disease, and other difficulties associated with menopause.

Dietary and Lifestyle Recommendations:

1. Eat the whole foods diet with an emphasis on plant foods, particularly fresh green leafy vegetables, tomatoes and carrots as well as whole grains.
2. Limit all forms of refined sugar.
3. Increase exercise, particularly if normally sedentary.

Nutritional Supplement Recommendations:

1. Vitamin C: 1,000-2,000 mg daily.
2. Beta-carotene: 150,000 IU daily. This requirement can be fulfilled by drinking carrot juice, without added pills or capsules.
3. Selenium: 400 mcg daily.
4. Zinc: 30 mg daily
5. Vitamin E: 400-800 IU daily.
6. Evening Primrose oil: 2 capsules twice daily, taken with vitamin E.
7. Vitex agnus-castus (chaste berry): 1-2 standardized capsules, or 40 drops of standardized liquid extract, each morning, to balance the hormones.
8. Follow the treatment suggestions under "Menorrhagia" and "Dysmenorrhea" in Part Four if needed.
9. Use a liver-supportive herb such as dandelion or milk thistle, to aid the body's natural detoxifying mechanism.

CHAPTER 2
OVARIAN CYSTS

Ovarian cysts are a part of the natural process of ovulation each month. As those four thousand single-cells in the ovary work to mature the one egg that is chosen, a fluid-filled follicle sac—a cyst—forms around the maturing egg. When the egg matures, the sac ruptures (bursts open) to release the egg for possible fertilization. When a woman feels the rupture that occurs, the pain she experiences is called *mittleschmerz*, a German word meaning "middle pain." Speedy healing occurs to the follicle, and the process is repeated the following month.

Abnormal Cysts:

Follicle Cysts

Some women, instead of merely producing these types of functional or simple cysts, may be predisposed to producing the cysts at other times, or of having a cyst remain for a few cycles before finally rupturing. I have had this happen myself, particularly while continuing to breastfeed my toddlers, when my cycles have not become completely fertile yet. A follicle cyst usually grows no larger than two inches in diameter, and requires no medical intervention, as it will eventually rupture—this can be painful. Following rupture, the cyst will shrink again, and the follicle heal. Many times, when I have gone to the doctor with unexplained pelvic pain, the bimanual vaginal exam itself is the catalyst for the rupture of the cyst. All that poking and prodding usually causes the cyst to rupture.

Any pain in the lower abdomen should be evaluated by a professional caregiver to rule out serious medical conditions.

Post-menopausal women with any type of cyst should be examined immediately, as the ovaries regress in size at menopause and should not be producing the cysts normally associated with the menstrual cycle.

Corpus Luteum Cysts

A corpus luteum cyst occurs when the normal corpus luteum, which is designed to produce progesterone to help sustain a pregnancy, becomes involute—that is, it does not decrease in size or progesterone production, but instead continues to grow past the time when menstruation should occur. These cysts are most common in the early part of pregnancy, although they can occur at other times. The pain and small amount of bleeding that occurs internally when they do rupture may simulate ectopic pregnancy. The reason for the pain is often the blood that irritates internal tissue. This can cause lingering pain for a few days after the ovarian cyst ruptures.

If a functional or corpus luteum cyst is found and evaluated, reevaluation should be done within two to four months, to make certain that either the cyst is gone or that it is not growing larger, which could indicate a need for further evaluation of the cyst.

Dermoid Cysts

Dermoid cysts make up about fifteen to twenty percent of abnormal ovarian growths. They can occur at any age, but account for about sixty percent of benign ovarian cysts in girls under age fifteen. Dermoid cysts are the second most common of all ovarian neoplasms— ovarian growths that grow to a large size, secrete hormones that alter normal physiologic functions: some neoplasms (not dermoid) can be malignant in women of any age group. Usually dermoid cysts are discovered when they are between five and ten centimeters in diameter, although they can grow to fifteen or more centimeters. About ten percent are bilateral—occurring in both ovaries. These tumors are the ones we all hear about that contain hair, skin, cartilage, and sometimes teeth. They generally require removal through surgery, since there is the possibility of malignancy occurring in an area of these otherwise benign ovarian cysts.

Dietary and Lifestyle Recommendations:

1. Emphasize a whole-foods diet, with plenty of fresh fruit and vegetables. Limit refined, processed foods.
2. Eliminate or limit caffeine-containing beverages.

3. High-quality protein works best for dealing with ovarian cysts: lean deep-sea fish, beans and grains.

4. If red meat and poultry are chosen, try to choose brands that are grown as naturally as possible to avoid any possible hormone residue in the tissue of the meat.

Nutritional Supplement Recommendations:

1. Aid the balancing of the hormones through use of vitex agnus-castus (chaste berry): 1-2 standardized capsules, or 40 drops of the standardized liquid extract, every morning throughout the month. This therapy may take several months to achieve hormonal balance.

2. A combination of the following herbs taken from the beginning of the menstrual flow until ovulation can be used for up to 9 months:
   - Blue cohosh root
   - Black cohosh root
   - Yarrow flower
   - Wild yam flower
   - Black haw bark
   - Milk thistle seed[1]

3. A combination of the following herbs taken from ovulation to the beginning of the next cycle's menstrual flow may be used:
   - chaste berry seed (vitex)
   - Black cohosh root
   - Dandelion root and leaf, equal parts
   - Wild yam root
   - Black haw bark[2]

4. For women who are perimenopausal (in the first stages of beginning menopause) or who desire one formula they can take all month, the following herbs may be used:
   - chaste berry seed (vitex)
   - Milk thistle seed
   - Wild yam root
   - Burdock root
   - Black cohosh root

CHAPTER 3
POLYCYSTIC OVARIAN SYNDROME (PCOS)

Polycystic ovarian syndrome (PCOS), also known as Stein-Leventhal syndrome, was first identified in 1905 as a syndrome consisting of amenorrhea, hirsutism and obesity in association with enlarged polycystic ovaries (ovaries having many cysts on them). Researchers now believe that the syndrome actually begins soon after the onset of menstruation in young girls. Some study authors refer to PCOS as a syndrome of hyperandrogenic chronic anovulation, as the ovaries of many women with PCOS are actually normal-sized, and women without PCOS may have polycystic ovaries. The focus of much of the current studies has not been on the ovaries of women with this syndrome but on the endocrine and hormonal aspects of the disease.

About three percent of teen girls and women have PCOS. An interesting factor is that women of different ethnic backgrounds exhibit different sets of symptoms. The symptoms most likely to be found with PCOS are:

* Lack of periods, or extremely irregular periods;
* Hirsutism: excessive facial and genital hair. Some women need to shave every day, while there may be thinning hair on the scalp;
* Apple-shaped figure due to weight gain: abdominal storage, rather than standard female thigh and waist storage (pear-shape);
* Insulin-resistance: hyperglycemia and/or hypoglycemia and/or diabetes and/or insulin level problems. This is a major feature of the disease on an endocrine level, and is now

thought perhaps to be causative of the entire syndrome. When insulin resistance is found along with high blood pressure, high triglyceride levels, decreased HDL (good cholesterol) and obesity, it is sometimes termed "Syndrome X;"

- Infertility: irregularity of ovulation reduces the odds of pregnancy each month. Endocrine problems may interfere with the mechanisms of conception, implantation and the first trimester of pregnancy;
- Ovarian cysts: ultrasound will show a honeycomb or "string of pearls" of partially developed follicles (eggs) coating the inside of the ovaries. As stated before, all women with PCOS do not experience problems with their ovaries at all;
- Painful ovulation: due to the enlargement and blockage of the surface of the ovaries;
- Dark velvety patches on the skin under the arms, breasts and nape of the neck;
- Adult acne;
- A mother or grandmother with some of these symptoms;
- A father or grandfather with premature (in his 20s) male pattern baldness.

What Tests are Done to Diagnose the Syndrome?

Ultrasound is generally used to check out the ovaries for cysts, but blood tests to check hormone levels are the best way to achieve an accurate diagnosis. Doctors look for high levels of androgens, particularly testosterone; high LH (luteinizing hormone) levels or an elevated LH to FSH (follicle stimulating hormone) ratio.

What Causes PCOS?

Most experts now believe that PCOS begins with the body becoming resistant to insulin, which leads to the release of more insulin to compensate for what the body is not assimilating. This condition is called hyperinsulinemia. The ovaries are very sensitive to this increased level of insulin, and start overproducing androgen hormones, such as testosterone. Since the ovaries are mass-producing testosterone, they do not signal the pituitary to lower LH levels, so the pituitary gland produces more LH, which leads to more production of testosterone. The follicles in the ovaries do not convert the testosterone to estrogen, which inhibits the normal development of a mature follicle, or egg, each month. Ovulation then does not take place because the ovary has no mature egg to release. The immature follicle becomes a tiny cyst that starts producing its own androgens, which further inhibits next month's follicle development and ovulation.

The androgens cause many of the symptoms of PCOS, but the root cause is the insulin resistance or hyperinsulinemia. The new treatment focus, both conventional and natural, is on enhancing insulin uptake.

What are the Problems and Risks Associated with PCOS?

Women with PCOS are at higher risk for developing a number of other health disorders. This risk does not mean it is inevitable that women with PCOS will develop these diseases; however, it does mean that women with PCOS have a higher risk than other women in the population for the following diseases:

* Type 2 Diabetes (adult-onset): this risk can be controlled through dietary changes and exercise. Untreated, the risk is up to forty percent of developing diabetes by age forty.
* High cholesterol and triglyceride levels: this risk too can be controlled through dietary changes and nutritional supplements.
* Cardiovascular disease: by controlling the two risks mentioned above, this risk can be greatly lowered.
* Endometrial cancer (cancer of the lining of the uterus): this risk results from lack of regular menstruation. I believe herbal medicine to be very effective in helping establish regular menstrual cycles.

Often, all of these risks can be controlled through the strategies listed below; however, any woman diagnosed with PCOS should be regularly seen by a physician as an essential part of her overall healthcare program. An herbalist/nutritionist should be a definite part of the conventional medical program for long-term preventive healthcare.

Dietary and Lifestyle Recommendations:

1. A whole foods diet is absolutely essential for this disorder, with an emphasis on high-fiber, high-complex carbohydrate foods to help control insulin levels. High-fiber, high-complex carbohydrates means eating: fresh fruits and vegetables, whole grains (not refined or processed), beans and legumes, with few or no sugar products and few animal products other than deep-sea fish, naturally-raised poultry, and red meat as a small portion on the plate.
2. Exercise is also an essential, as exercise is a very effective way of controlling insulin levels. Walking is an effective exercise and can be fairly enjoyable if done where one is comfortable.
3. If you are already experiencing problems with insulin control, or have diabetes, a completely vegan diet has been shown to reduce the risk of health conditions associated with diabetes. A vegan diet is entirely made up of plant foods, with no animal foods whatsoever.
4. Olive oil should be used instead of margarine or butter. Olive oil has a protective effect against heart disease.
5. Dairy products should probably be avoided, as current research indicates that there is an increased incidence of diabetes in those who drink milk.

6. Smoking should be avoided.
7. Moderate alcohol consumption in healthy people is actually good for the health, but in a high-risk person, as with animal foods, it is probably best avoided.

Nutritional Supplement Recommendations:

The following are recommended to deal with insulin resistance. There are combination supplements on the market that will likely contain a number of the following nutrients and herbs for insulin resistance:

1. Vitamin E: 900 IU daily.
2. Vitamin C: 1,000 mg to a maximum of 3,000 mg daily.
3. Vitamin B_6: 1,800 mg daily of a special form of vitamin B_6 has improved glucose tolerance dramatically in some research.[1]
4. Biotin: 16 mg daily
5. Vitamin B_3, niacin: 500-750 mg per day for 1 month, followed with a maintenance dosage of 250mg per day. If flushing occurs, reduce the dosage.
6. Chromium: 200 mcg daily.
7. Magnesium: 300-400 mg daily.
8. Zinc: 15-25 mg per day.
9. Coenzyme Q_{10}: 120 mg per day may be helpful, although the research is not clear at this point that it definitely is helpful.
10. Inositol: 500 mg taken twice each day.
11. Carnitine: 1 mg per 2.2 pounds of body weight each day. One trial showed that both cholesterol and triglyceride levels dropped 25-39% in just 10 days.[2]
12. Gymnema herb may assist the pancreas in the production of insulin: 400 mg daily of gymnema extract.
13. Panax ginseng at a dosage of 200 mg daily has improved blood glucose level control as well as energy levels in those with insulin-resistance.[3]
14. Aloe vera juice: 1 tablespoon twice daily can help lower blood sugar levels.[4]
15. Bitter melon (whole, fried slices[5], water extracts[6] and juice[7]) may improve blood sugar control in Type 2 diabetics.

To deal with the hormonal imbalance:

1. Vitex agnus-castus (chaste berry): vitex is known for its effect on lowering LH levels in an effort to balance hormonal function, as well as for its ability to establish regular menstrual cycles. Take 1-2 capsules or 40 drops of the standardized extract each morning. This therapy may take 3-6 months to regulate the cycles.
2. Saw palmetto extract has been shown in studies to lower excess testosterone levels, thus would be a good herb to use for PCOS.

CHAPTER 4:
CERVICAL DYSPLASIA

Cervical dysplasia means abnormal, or dysfunctional, cell growth on the cervix. Having cervical dysplasia does not mean a woman has cervical cancer. There are certainly benign conditions that can cause a diagnosis of cervical dysplasia, such as:

❋ chronic cervicitis, which is chronic inflammation of the cervix

❋ hyperplasia: refers to cells that are growing a bit too fast and too thick. This can occur because of the cervix trying to protect itself from physical injury or chemical irritation. I had a polyp grow on one side of my cervix following a cervical laceration during childbirth. My polyp would be termed hyperplasia yet was not cancerous in the least

❋ neoplasia is a term used for new cell growth, which can be cancerous but is not definitive for cancer.

A word about "cervical erosion:" Cervical erosion occurs after a sustained period of either: untreated vaginitis (a vaginal infection that is keeping the cervix regularly inflamed); inflammation from chemicals used in the vagina (perhaps from contraceptive foams, gels, suppositories or tampons containing chemicals); or from physical inflammatory processes, such as repeated injury to the cervix. Over time, the cells (epithelial) that line the cervical os (the internal portion of the cervix) start to turn outward onto the downward-facing surface of the cervix. These cells are not designed to handle physical irritation, so they become inflamed and lead to the cervix becoming painful, perhaps spotting after intercourse or the physical stresses mentioned above. As the inflammation increases, new cells will grow as others are sloughed off, and the new cells are not always healthy cells. The fragile surface of the cervix where the epithelial cells are in the wrong place and getting damaged is called "cervical erosion."

If all the cells do not grow into normal, healthy cells, cervical dysplasia results where there is a presence of abnormal cells lining the cervix. These patches of abnormal cells lining the surface of the cervix then are called "squamous intrapithelial cells" (SIL). While cervical dysplasia is thought to be one of the first steps in the development of cancer, studies show that low-grade dysplasia often regresses on its own, with absolutely no intervention. Since we are concerned here with working with our body's natural processes and function to increase the health of our new cells, we will address the various "grades" of dysplasia, some of the current thinking a major cause of dysplasia, as well as the nutritional interventions we might employ to help our body return to producing healthy, normal cells in our cervix.

What does an "abnormal result" actually mean?

Since approximately two to five percent of Pap smears will have an abnormal result, the first thing we need to do is understand what that abnormal result actually means. The usual abnormal result categories are:

❀ atypical cells of uncertain significance (ASCUS): this means "we don't know why you have atypical cells; we will keep a watch on them."

❀ mild dysplasia, or low-grade squamous intraepithelial neoplasia (LGSIL)

❀ moderate to severe dysplasia, or high-grade squamous intraepithelial neoplasia (HGSIL)

Since cervical cancer usually grows quite slowly over a period of years without invading nearby tissue, we usually have some time to work naturally with abnormal results that in most cases regress on their own. A study that is helpful to our understanding of how cervical dysplasia progresses (or not) is a 1998 study[1] that looked at all scientific studies in the medical literature since 1970 in which women with abnormal Pap smears were followed but not treated. They analyzed how often the Pap smear results improved with no intervention and how often the results progressed to a worsening lesion or grade of abnormality.

Abnormal Pap Smear: Natural Progression and Regression

ABNORMAL CLASS	REGRESSION TO NORMAL	PROGRESSION TO HIGHER GRADE OVER 24 MONTHS	PROGRESSION TO INVASIVE CANCER OVER 24 MONTHS
ASCUS	68%	7%	0.25%
LGSIL	47%	21%	0.15%
HGSIL	35%	23%	1.44%

As you can see, in the majority of cases, the abnormal cell findings regressed on their own, even in high-grade dysplasia. I feel this gives most women time to embark on a natural course of therapy while continuing with follow-ups with their physician. In fact, one naturopathic physician, Tori Hudson, N.D., completed a very successful study funded by the National Institutes of Health (NIH) on natural treatments for cervical dysplasia. Her results were highly satisfactory and may be considered as an alternative to conventional medical treatment for dysplasia—a condition that, in and of itself, is NOT cancerous—which is, typically, to freeze or burn off the abnormal cells, possibly causing more abnormal cellular growth through more injury to the cervix. Dr. Hudson's therapy will be discussed under "Recommendations."

What will my doctor want to do with my dysplasia results?

If you have an abnormal pap smear result, your doctor will want to look at your cervix with a device called a colposcope—a powerful magnifying glass that looks somewhat like a pair of binoculars mounted on a stand. If your doctor sees areas of dysplasia, she will take a very small biopsy to confirm the diagnosis. If the results of the biopsy confirm that dysplasia is present, your doctor should give you several options for therapy:

1. Observation: In many instances, the mild dysplasia will go away on its own. If, over time, the mild dysplasia worsens to moderate or severe dysplasia, then the abnormal cells can be treated at that time, if you choose.

2. Cryotherapy: Cryotherapy is the medical term for freezing therapy of the cervix. A small metal disc, approximately half an inch in diameter, is placed against the cervix. The disc is attached to a device that can produce extreme cold, freezing the outermost cells of the cervix. This freezing destroys the dysplasia cells, thus, it is hoped, allowing normal cells to

heal in their place. Cryotherapy can be performed in the doctor's office, takes about ten minutes, and may cause minor cramping. It also results in a watery discharge from the vagina for approximately eight weeks following therapy.

3. Laser Therapy: A small laser can be used to destroy the outermost cells of the cervix, in much the same way that cryotherapy freezes these cells. After the dysplasia cells have been vaporized by the laser, normal cells heal back in their place. Laser therapy takes only a few minutes. Although it may cause cramping, it has almost no other side effects. However, the laser is very expensive, and sometimes the procedure must be performed either in a hospital or an outpatient surgery center.

4. Loop Electrosurgical Excision Procedure (LEEP): Sometimes referred to simply as a "loop" procedure, LEEP uses a small loop of wire through which electricity is passed, which produces a cutting effect in tissue. With this cutting wire loop, the area of dysplasia can be surgically excised, allowing normal tissue to heal back in its place. Excision using the wire loop does not produce any pain in the cervix, and the whole procedure is minimally uncomfortable. The wire loop is sometimes used to remove more tissue than is usually destroyed with cryotherapy or laser therapy.

Any of the treatments from 2 to 4 above can have an effect on childbearing and general cervical health. Since even high-grade cervical dysplasias (SILs) take years (ten to fifteen, according to the National Cancer Institute) to progress to cervical cancer, it seems a bit too aggressive to elect immediately for one of these procedures at the first hint of dysplasia. Perhaps a reasonable time period of aggressive natural therapy is warranted before taking steps that damage the cervix even more.

There ARE instances where dysplasia is associated with conditions that cause cancer to come on more quickly. The significant factor is human papilloma virus (HPV).

Human papilloma virus (HPV)

Human papilloma virus (HPV) is the cause of genital warts, the most common viral sexually-transmitted disease. Genital warts are small, flat or mushroom-shaped growths that may appear singly or in clusters on the genitals of women and men. They are not usually painful, and only thirty percent of those infected actually develop visible warts; seventy percent of HPV-infected individuals never develop warts. Obviously, then, there is a great number of people who do not know that they are infected. HPV has been found to be a major causative factor in cervical dysplasia and cervical cancer. The virus is transmitted through the skin, usually during sexual intercourse, although it may not always be sexually-transmitted. It is estimated that as many as five to twenty percent of persons fifteen to forty-nine years of age are infected with HPV.

Certain strains of HPV, types HPV-16, HPV-18, HPV-31, and HPV-45, are high risk. They account for eighty percent of cervical cancer. How does HPV affect the progression of an abnormal Pap smear? In one study, the rate of progression of cervical dysplasia was higher with HPV (50.5%) than without HPV (35.4%). Of the cases with HPV that progressed, HPV-16 progressed at a rate of 56.5%, while those with HPV-6 and/or 11, only 30.8% progressed. Therefore, the type of HPV matters in terms of likelihood of progression to higher-grade dysplasia and cervical cancer.[2] Another study in 1987 looked at progression or regression of a Pap smear showing HPV-compatible changes.[3]

Abnormal Class	Regression to Normal	Progression to Higher Grade Over 24 Months	Progression to Invasive Cancer Over 24 Months
HPV only	45%	16%	0%
HPV and LGSIL		50%	0%

If I have a pap smear that shows HPV, do I have a sexually-transmitted disease?

If it was your Pap smear or a biopsy that was read as HPV changes, then it is only about eighty-five percent accurate. Cytotechnologists look for what is called koilocytosis: if it is seen, it is called HPV-compatible. Viral cultures or smears for HPV fragments are the more certain way to diagnose HPV; therefore, it would seem prudent for monogamous women to have the viral culture or smear to diagnose HPV, rather than relying on their Pap smear results alone. HPV can be latent for many years; thus, a woman may have contracted the disease at a much earlier date and only be diagnosed later in life.

Dietary and Lifestyle Recommendations:

1. Since making healthy cells is so important for this condition, it seems advisable to be very diligent in providing our body with plenty of good, whole foods to eat, with very little processed or refined foods that will not supply potent nutrient content. Fresh fruit and vegetables should be eaten freely throughout the day to supply our bodies with live enzymes for healing.
2. Eliminate sources of injury to the cervix:
   ❀ don't use tampons and vaginal contraceptives;

- ❀ be gentle during intercourse, particularly if intercourse is painful or causes spotting afterwards;
- ❀ be careful during childbirth to limit injury to the cervix;
- ❀ don't introduce objects into the vagina that don't naturally belong there (this does not include your husband!).

Nutritional Supplement Recommendations:

1. Immune system support through herbs such as:
   - ❀ garlic: the equivalent of 1 clove, 3 times daily
   - ❀ echinacea: 500-1,000 mg twice daily
   - ❀ vitamin A: 50,000 IU daily for 2 months, then 25,000 IU daily (if no abnormal liver function is in your health history)
   - ❀ vitamin C and bioflavonoids: 2,500 mg daily
   - ❀ vitamin E: 800 IU daily
   - ❀ zinc: 30 mg daily
   - ❀ folic acid: 5 mg twice a day for 3 months, then 2.5 mg daily
   - ❀ selenium: 400 mcg daily
   - ❀ germanium : 30 mg GE daily
   - ❀ flaxseed oil may be taken to enhance immune function: 1 tablespoon twice daily.

2. Herbal formula consisting of: dandelion, licorice, goldenseal and red clover taken twice daily for three months.

3. Vaginal topical protocol #1:
   - ❀ Week One: Dr. Tori Hudson's "Vita A" vitamin A suppository nightly for six nights.
   - ❀ Week Two: Dr. Hudson's "Herbal-C" herbal vaginal suppository nightly for six nights, containing myrrh, echinacea, usnea, goldenseal, marshmallow, geranium and yarrow.
   - ❀ Week 3: "Vita A" nightly for six nights.
   - ❀ Week 4: "Herbal C" nightly for six nights.

4. After that four-week protocol, switch to vaginal protocol #2:
   Week 1: "Vita-A" nightly for six nights plus
   One vaginal depletion pack with vitamin A or two "Vag Pack" suppositories done once weekly
   Week 2: "Herbal-C" nightly for six nights plus
   Same as week 1
   Week 3: "Vita-A" nightly for six nights plus
   Same as week 1

Week 4: "Herbal-C" nightly for six nights plus
Same as week 1

Vaginal Depletion Pack:

$MgSO_4$ (anhydrous magnesium sulfate)	8 ounces
Glycerin (same as vegetable glycerin, glycerol)	4-6 ounces
Tea tree essential oil	1 ounce
Thuja essential oil	½ ounce
Bitter orange oil	¼ ounce
Goldenseal tincture	½ ounce
Vita Minerals 120 (iron sulfate solution)	1 ounce

1. Pour the $MgSO_4$ into a wide-mouthed 16-ounce glass container (with tight-fitting lid) until it is half full.
2. Add glycerin until soupy.
3. Mix vigorously after each of the following steps, or the solution will not be usable.
4. Add essential oils.
5. Add goldenseal tincture.
6. Add Vita Minerals 120.

Stir occasionally over the next 2 or 3 hours, until the mixture has a thick, tar-like consistency. Store in a tightly sealed container in a cool place (50-70 degrees is ideal). Stir once a week if you are not using it regularly. This mixture will keep indefinitely with proper storage and occasional stirring.

TO USE: Fold a piece of cotton cloth (1/2 by 2 by 3 inches long) lengthwise into a tube. Tie one end with a 4 inch cotton string or dental floss, leaving a long tail. Put 1 tablespoon of the formula into the untied end of the cotton tube. Using a speculum (the disposable speculum you bought for 1 or 2 dollars from a birth-supplier will work just fine), expose the cervix, open the speculum wide enough to insert the pack and slide the pack, formula-end first, tightly up against the cervix. Leave the string exposed for later removal of the herb pack. Leave the pack in for twenty-four hours, then remove it by pulling the string. Follow with a mild apple-cider vinegar douche (1 teaspoon of vinegar diluted in 8 ounces of water).

Women will notice increased vaginal drainage with use. If a burning sensation occurs in the vagina, remove the pack immediately and follow with the apple-cider douche. The cervix will have a red appearance where old cells are sloughing off; this will heal in 7-10 days. Do not schedule Pap smears until at least 10 days after application of the Vaginal Depletion Pack. It may be best to wait at least 3 months before a follow-up Pap smear, to allow time for the natural therapy to begin working and healing.

CHAPTER 5:
ENDOMETRIOSIS

Endometriosis is a condition in which the lining of the uterus, which naturally builds up and thickens to provide the home into which a newly conceived baby will implant, allows its cells to travel outside the uterus and continue their monthly cycle of build-up and bleeding according to hormonal influence. These traveling cells of the endometrium attach themselves to other areas, most commonly the cervix, ovaries, fallopian tubes, bladder or intestines, although they have been known to travel much further into other areas of the body, wreaking havoc.

Approximately five percent of American women have endometriosis. Symptoms include severe menstrual cramps, excessive bleeding, gas, pain during ovulation or intercourse, leading sometimes to depression and insomnia. A recent German study found that women between twenty and twenty-nine years of age being treated for endometriosis reported menstrual pain (90%); infertility (80%), pelvic pain (71%) and menstrual irregularity (46%). The bleeding that occurs outside the uterus can lead to scarring and inflammation of the organs to which the aberrant tissue has attached itself. Blood from the tissue can form "chocolate cysts," which are quite painful when they burst. The prognosis for fertility in women with endometriosis is only fifty percent, making this both a physically and emotionally painful disorder.

Risk Factors

We simply do not know what causes endometriosis, although some clues point to an excess of estrogen. We do know that women who do not bear children in their early years are more likely to have endometriosis. This is another instance where we see that our female bodies are designed for early marriage and early childbearing, rather than for our cultural norm of waiting until we have our careers firmly established before pursuing marriage and family.

The Environmental Protection Agency (EPA) linked endometriosis and dioxin levels in several studies on female monkeys in 1994. These monkeys developed endometriosis when exposed to dioxin. The chemical structure of dioxin, some polychlorinated biphenyls (PCBs), and some pesticides, mimic human estrogen, and are stored, as estrogen is, in human fatty tissue. Another study found that women who drink alcohol have a fifty percent higher risk of developing endometriosis than those who abstain, although the study results do not indicate whether moderate alcohol consumption has the same risk factors.

Usual Treatment Protocol

Physicians generally treat with
- ❀ surgery
- ❀ Danazol, a drug with so many negative side effects that I don't believe it should continue to be offered
- ❀ GnRH (gonadotropin-releasing hormone) analogs, which are synthesized versions of GnRH. These should not be used for more than six months, according to the FDA guidelines
- ❀ progesterone, primarily in the form of Depo-Provera (a long-acting contraceptive) or oral Provera (synthetic progesterone which increases one's risk of reproductive cancers)
- ❀ estrogen/progesterone (oral contraceptive), the treatment of choice among doctors.

Dietary and Lifestyle Recommendations:

1. As in every other health concern, switch to and maintain a whole-foods diet. Make certain you are getting fresh fruit and vegetables each day. This cannot be emphasized enough for overall health.
2. Exercise to increase circulation, although don't go on a major exercise campaign, which can lead to a worsening of symptoms. Ease into your exercise program, just as you eased yourself into more whole foods.
3. A diet low in animal fat, as well as an overall low-fat diet, is in order, to decrease excess estrogen.
4. Follow the recommendations for PMS, as that entire protocol is geared toward lowering excess estrogen levels.
5. Eliminate cigarettes, and any excess of 3 glasses of wine each week.
6. Use sanitary pads instead of tampons, which can "stop up" the menstrual flow.

7. Follow the recommendations under "Dysmenorrhea" for the pain during menstruation.
8. Eliminate caffeine.

Nutritional Supplement Recommendations:

1. Use phytoestrogenic herbs, such as soy, red clover and black cohosh to fill estrogen receptor-sites, thus not allowing excess estrogen to fill up the sites causing problems. I really like a formula called Equilibrium by NF Formulas for reducing pain and providing daily phytoestrogens for women with endometriosis and perimenopausal women.
2. Black haw bark is a potent antispasmodic for the uterus. Other antispasmodics that can be used are: cramp bark, valerian, chamomile and wild yam.
3. Saw palmetto extract can be useful in this condition for its anti-inflammatory effect as well as reducing excess testosterone levels. 2 capsules in the morning and one in the evening.
4. Flaxseed oil may be used at 1 tablespoon twice daily.
5. Red raspberry leaf may be used as a uterine tonic. 2 capsules twice daily or 3 cups of the tea daily.
6. Grape seed extract or muscadine grape seed extract are potent antioxidants containing anthocyanadins that give healing to connnective tissue. 1-3 tablets or capsules may be taken daily.
7. Red root may be used to encourage lymphatic cleansing. The lymph system is responsible for helping the body to remove toxins and infectious material.
8. Liver-supportive herbs such as burdock, dandelion, yellow dock and milk thistle are indicated. Choose one of these or a combination of them for use with meals.
9. Vitex agnus-castus (chaste berry) is definitely indicated for hormonal imbalance of any kind: 1 capsule or tablet of the standardized formula, or 40 drops of the standardized liquid extract, taken each morning.
10. Evening Primrose oil, black currant or borage seed oil provide for anti-inflammatory action that may be helpful for women with endometriosis. Take as directed on bottle.

Chapter 6
Benign Breast Disease

Fibrocystic Breast Disease, sometimes called cystic mastitis or benign breast lumps, is a sometimes painful, although benign, cystic swelling of the breasts. The pain or tenderness tends to occur prior to menstruation or after gaining weight. The term disease is really unfair and scary. It is a set of symptoms that commonly occur in healthy women (lumpy, swollen breasts with sometime nipple discharge) and is NOT a precursor to breast cancer.[1] The cysts, which may be quite small or large, are fluid-filled sacs that are not cancerous. These lumps naturally diminish after menopause.

Fluctuating estrogen levels may aggravate the condition, as well as caffeine in coffee, teas and colas, theophylline in tea and theobromine in chocolate. Infrequent bowel movements may also have a direct bearing on cystic mastitis. Women who have fewer than three bowel movements per week are more likely to have this condition. This may be due to reabsorption of estrogens that the liver has sent to be eliminated through the bowels.

There are other types of benign breast tumors that we will mention here as they may show up on a mammogram, creating a need to know.

What are benign breast conditions?

The two main types of tissue in the breast, glandular (the lobules and ducts of the breasts) and stromal (the fatty tissue and supporting ligaments) can undergo changes that cause diseases or disorders. The most common of benign breast conditions include:

1. Fibrocystic changes (discussed above)
2. Benign breast tumors:
    - The most common is the fibroadenoma, seen in women under age 40 and occasionally in teens. Fibroadenomas are usually round with distinct borders, can be several centimeters across and are movable under the skin. The only way to identify them accurately is through biopsy, which is recommended for any woman over 20 with a suspicious breast tumor that is growing. It is extremely rare for a fibroadenoma to develop cancerous areas within the benign tumor.
    - Nipple adenomas occur in the nipple area. They can vary in their appearance, sometimes recurring after removal, and are only rarely associated with cancer.
    - Intraductal papillomas are relatively uncommon small growths that line the milk ducts near the nipple. These benign breast tumors are usually seen in women over 40, and usually produce a discharge, which may be bloody.

Any breast lump should be evaluated by your physician and by mammogram.

3. Breast inflammation, which most commonly occurs during breastfeeding from plugged ducts. Plugged ducts, if left untreated, can lead to mastitis (breast infection). We treat plugged ducts, seen as a hard, red area on the affected breast, by breastfeeding often on that side. Rest is imperative, as is taking vitamin C and echinacea every 2 hours, while drinking at least 2 quarts of water daily.

Treatment for benign breast conditions is usually based on overall health and medical history, extent of the problem, your tolerance for specific medications, procedures or therapies, expectations for the course of the disease as well as your preference for treatment. At best, dietary changes may be implemented. At worst, minor surgical procedures to biopsy or remove the tumor may be necessary (see Part Two, Chapter 2: Routine Testing).

Lifestyle and Dietary Recommendations:

1. Consume plenty of fruits and vegetables. Eat more plant-based proteins, rather than meat, to encourage regular bowel movements. Animal fat may contribute to the growth of cysts. A strong link between fat and symptoms has been noted, thus more of a plant-based diet is indicated for this condition.
2. Eliminate coffee, tea, chocolate and caffeinated sodas.
3. Eat deep-sea fish or sea vegetables rich in iodine.
4. Do regular breast self-exams and alert your healthcare provider to any new lumps.

5. Rule out a possible wheat allergy by eliminating all wheat products for 2 weeks, then reintroducing wheat to see if allergy symptoms develop.

Nutritional Supplement Recommendations:

1. Vitamin E: 400-600 IU daily.
2. Beta-carotene: 10,000-25,000 IU daily.
3. Evening Primrose oil has been used successfully in Europe to reduce the size of cysts.[2] Take 1-2 capsules 3 times daily.
4. Gotu kola has been clinically documented as an effective treatment for fibrocystic breast disease.[3] 500 to 1,000 mg daily.
5. Vitamin B_6: 50 - 200mg in a B-complex of other B vitamins in 25 mg amounts.
6. Magnesium: 200 mg daily.
7. Zinc: 10-40 mg daily.
8. Cold-pressed flaxseed oil: 1-2 tablespoons daily.
9. Vitamin C: 60 mg daily.
10. Iodine from sea kelp, either as food, or 4-6 capsules daily.
11. Vitex agnus-castus (chaste berry) may be used each morning to help balance the female hormones. Take 1-2 standardized tablets or capsules, or 40 drops of the standardized liquid extract.
12. Castor oil packs may be of benefit, used 3-4 times weekly for up to 6 months. Saturate a flannel cloth with castor oil (I prefer the odorless castor oil found in pharmacies) and heat it in a 350° oven until warm. Place the pack over the breast and cover it with plastic food wrap or a small towel to keep it warm. The skin will absorb the castor oil's active constituents, lectins, which stimulate a local immune response, act as an analgesic, and as an anti-inflammatory agent.
13. Place cabbage leaves inside the bra to relieve the pain and swelling associated with breast inflammation. I know this sounds weird, but we use it all the time in women with plugged ducts or breast infections with great success.

CHAPTER 7
ABNORMAL MAMMOGRAMS

Although we have addressed going for a mammogram in Part Two under Routine Testing, we will here address what happens when the results come back with an indication for further testing. The mere fact of having to go in for a mammogram is a potent reminder of the possibility of breast cancer. Many women never make it in for a mammogram because of their fear of what they might find. I know that even I, with a family history of early-onset breast cancer, waited until I was thirty-three to get a baseline, and would not have gone even then if I had not seen a friend with a similar family history be diagnosed with breast cancer herself. The stress level is usually quite high over mammogram results, particularly when there is anything more than "The radiologist finds nothing that causes a concern for breast cancer."

What do mammogram results actually mean?

The important thing to remember is that there are many cases when the screening will show an area of abnormality without that abnormality being classified as possible cancer. The American College of Radiology has five categories for classifying mammography results:

1. A finding of "0" means that the mammogram needs to be redone, because the quality of the pictures was not adequate. This can happen if all of the breast was not placed within the x-ray field. This is why I prefer to endure a bit of discomfort to get a flatter breast on the plates, rather than having to redo the results. Any redo increases stress levels.

2. A "1" is what every woman wants: negative.

3. A "2" indicates the identification of an abnormality, but one that is clearly benign or not harmful. These abnormalities are things like calcium, in benign growths called fibroadenomas. Many times this result will mean a follow-up diagnostic ultrasound to see if the abnormality is a benign fluid-filled cyst or solid, and, if solid, to see if the borders are well-defined, as in fibroadenomas.

4. A "3" is much like "2" above, an abnormality that is very likely benign. Still, there is a slight doubt. Rather than subjecting the woman to a biopsy right off the bat, a repeat mammography at a short interval, 3-6 months, is scheduled. What the doctors will look for is changes in the area in question. A harmless or benign tumor will have little or no change in this time period. A cancer will likely have noticeable growth and change. If there is significant change, the doctor will likely schedule a biopsy to better evaluate what the area may be. While most women will be asked to wait the short interval to check for changes, if there is a family history of breast cancer or if a woman is considered high risk, she will more than likely be referred for biopsy right away. This does not indicate that everyone assumes it is cancer; rather, an aggressive approach will better serve a woman who will spend the next few months worrying over what might be.

5. Even "4" is merely suspicious of cancer. Immediate biopsies are considered at this level, but not always. Again, your family history and risk factors weigh heavily here, as well as pictures that are not absolutely clear. This is what occurred with me. My tumor was found so close to my chest wall that it was hard to capture; the borders were not well-defined on the x-ray pictures. Because of this, and my family history, a biopsy was scheduled immediately.

6. Only level "5" is considered a high chance of cancer. In these cases, it is treated as though it is cancer, until shown to be otherwise.

Repeat testing at a short interval is a common response to slightly abnormal screening test results that have a low chance of being serious. This is the same response when dealing with abnormal Pap smear results. This is done primarily to prevent needless, interventive testing. While I agree with this plan in general, I do believe that every woman should have the option of further testing at the time when an abnormality is discovered, if she has a serious concern about the possibility of cancer. We live in our skin and know what is normal for us. If we are experiencing symptoms that concern us, we need to be listened to and treated accordingly by our professional caregivers. The importance of this attitude among women is illustrated by the personal story of my good friend, Robin Fergon, which appears at the end of this chapter.

What are the signs and symptoms of breast cancer?

Although there are many signs that are associated with being suspicious for breast cancer, the following symptoms definitely need to be further evaluated by your physician:

* breast masses that are firm, non-tender, irregular, without distinct borders, that are not movable and/or fixed to the skin or underlying muscle
* skin dimpling
* nipple retraction
* redness
* an orange-peel skin texture (where you have many small dimples on the outer skin)
* nipple discharge in only one breast, especially bloody discharge (found particularly in older women, but my grandmother had this in her 30s, and I have experienced this myself; my grandmother's discharge required the removal of half of one of her breasts, while my own showed no sign of further problem in my breast—it's a case of watch and see). Once again, I must say that sometimes we have to be bold in requesting care. Even after removal of a suspicious (turned out benign) tumor in one breast, when I had bloody discharge from the nipple in that same breast not even 6 months later, my physician was busy when I saw her, and concentrating on my pregnancy concerns. I had to ask her to look at the discharge, and had to, again, ask her nurse before leaving the office what we were going to do about this new occurrence. Be diligent! Keep pursuing!
* enlarged lymph nodes in the neck or under the arm. This is less common as the first sign of breast cancer. More often than not, we need to first evaluate whether these enlarged lymph nodes are caused by an infectious process in our upper respiratory tract or skin, a very common cause of enlarged lymph nodes in the neck. Any enlargement, though, that continues for more than 2 weeks, should be further evaluated by a physician.

Where Does Breast Cancer Generally Occur?

The most common site of breast cancer is the upper outer quadrant, where most of the breast tissue is located. In practical terms, that means the area closest to the armpit. Approximately 50% of breast cancers occur in this area. The upper inner quadrant is associated with a 15% incidence, while the lower outer and lower inner quadrants are associated with an 11% and 6% incidence, respectively. The central region, the area of the nipple and areola, is associated with 17% of breast cancers. While we may want to think that we don't need to worry about any of the above signs in an area of the breast that is less likely to have breast cancer occur, this seems unwise, as malignancy in the breast tissue can occur anywhere in the breast. Any change in the normal texture of the breast skin or feel of tissue in the breast should be noted in your breast self-exam, and talked over with your physician.

What happens if my mammogram results require further testing?

The first step is usually a diagnostic ultrasound. Ultrasonography uses high-energy sound waves that can pass through the breast. This can show whether a lump is solid or filled with fluid. Having an ultrasound on the breast is not in the least uncomfortable or painful. The nice thing about a follow-up mammogram and diagnostic ultrasound is that there is no waiting for results. The radiologist will report directly to you, to give you the results as soon as the test is completed.

If the abnormality is solid and suspicious in the least, the radiologist may recommend a biopsy to determine whether there are any malignant cells within the tumor. Biopsy may be done in several ways:

● Aspiration or fine-needle biopsy: the doctor uses a needle to remove fluid or a small amount of tissue from the breast. This procedure may show whether a lump is a fluid-filled cyst or a solid lump (which may or may not be cancerous). The tissue goes to a pathology lab to be checked for cancer cells. The drawback of this procedure is that it may miss an area of the tumor that is growing malignant cells. This is the least interventive method of further evaluation.

● Surgical biopsy: a surgeon cuts out part of a lump or suspicious area. This tissue is also sent to a pathologist to be examined under a microscope to check for cancer cells. This area is often marked for the surgeon by a special type of mammography or ultrasonography, called a needle localization. A wire is inserted into an abnormal area of the breast, using a local anesthetic to the breast. The patient is then sent to the operating room with the wire in place. This maps out the exact area of the breast that the surgeon should remove. The most uncomfortable portion of the needle localization is the compression on the breast to get it ready for the radiologist to insert the needle. Also, if there is a wait for a surgical suite, one must remain still to avoid dislodging the needle, which can make for an uncomfortable wait for surgery.

● Lumpectomy: Although many surgeons do not choose this method, I found it to be my procedure of choice with my own breast tumor. I couldn't see a reason why I would want to go through surgery, only to find I needed yet another surgery to remove the lump or my breast. I chose to have the whole thing removed. Now, I don't have any further worry, and the procedure was no more invasive than a surgical biopsy.

● A new device was approved in 1999 by the FDA to determine whether a woman needs a biopsy, the T-Scan 2000. The T-Scan 2000 is a handheld scan probe that is placed on the breast to evaluate suspicious areas of abnormality as detected on a mammogram. The probe is connected to a computer, which displays an image of those areas of the breast. The T-Scan images are based on measuring the differences in the electrical flow between malignant tumor tissue and the surrounding normal tissue. Areas with possible malignancy contain bright spots on the image projected on the computer. Concerns over how the device will handle the hormonal changes during the menstrual cycle, and its ability to detect and distinguish breast abnormalities, are still being discussed.

A PERSONAL STORY
BY ROBIN FERGON, BREAST CANCER SURVIVOR

I don't know if you are anything like me, but often I check my brain "out to lunch" when visiting my healthcare practitioner. Yes, I do go in with a list of questions, but frequently they are not answered sufficiently, or I am so nervous that I hear what I want to hear and don't hear what I should hear.

What is our responsibility concerning our own health, and where does the healthcare practitioner fit into the realm of things?

In November 1998, I made an appointment with a local breast care center for a diagnostic mammogram. With this type of appointment, you have the mammogram, and then the radiologist goes over the film, examines you, and makes recommendations for further evaluation if necessary. I made this particular appointment because of a lump I had discovered in my breast during a routine monthly breast self-exam. I also had seen dimpling in the breast when I raised my arm over my head, which can be another red flag for breast cancer. Both my grandmother and mother have had breast cancer, so this definitely added to my concern about the situation.

It was easier not to face the possibility of a tumor...

A small marker was placed over the lump, to assist the radiologist in pinpointing the area of complaint. After the mammogram was completed, the radiologist came in and examined me and said that nothing suspicious was found. I was told to come back in one year. I went flying out of the office, feeling grateful that this scare was over, and didn't give it another thought for several weeks. However, it was not long before I had this nagging feeling that all was not well. I reminded myself that I had had it checked out by a reputable doctor, and decided I needed to trust his expertise in his area of study. I did not want to face the possibility that it could be a tumor, so it was easier for me to ignore that nagging suspicion that all might *not* be well.

Eight months later, I decided to pursue that nagging suspicion. I had another mammogram, and requested an ultrasound. This showed a solid, two centimeter tumor. A week later, a surgeon confirmed my suspicion of a malignant tumor, and we discussed options for treatment.

In the year or so since my diagnosis, I have undergone surgery for removal of the tumor, two additional surgeries for complications from a staph infection, three months of chemotherapy, and two surgeries for the placement and removal of a port-a-cath for the administration of chemotherapy. I am very grateful that my treatment is complete and I can once again return to the many activities that I enjoy doing as a wife and mother.

Could things have been different?

I have had some time to reflect on events of the past year. I have asked myself if the outcome would have been different had I pursued that nagging feeling a little sooner, or had asked for an ultrasound during the initial diagnostic mammogram, or if I had had a different radiologist. Perhaps a proper diagnosis could have been made months earlier.

So what *is* a patient's responsibility in managing her own health? Having a strong family history of breast cancer, it was my responsibility to make sure that I maintained a routine of monthly breast self-exams, to know the signs of possible breast cancer, and to have routine exams and diagnostic testing as deemed necessary. Knowing what is involved in these routine exams and testing, and knowing what certain protocols are involved, can certainly make a difference in an accurate diagnosis. My case was a perfect example of this: with a palpable lump in my breast, and a negative mammogram, I should have insisted on an ultrasound. And, if that were still negative, I should have investigated the possibility of a biopsy.

It is tremendously important to find a reputable facility for diagnostic testing, and a doctor in whom you feel confident. Don't forget that you have the option of requesting a second opinion, especially if you feel that your questions have not been answered thoroughly.

While in the hospital, it is helpful, and sometimes necessary, for someone to stay with you at all times. I had several friends take turns staying with me while my husband was at work during the day. This turned out to be a wise plan, because on two occasions I was given the wrong medication. This may have been quite serious had the error not been caught. Unfortunately, nurses are overworked, and many medical facilities are understaffed, which causes a higher incidence of errors to occur.

Making a list of questions and concerns can also be very helpful. Prior to beginning chemotherapy, I had an appointment with my oncologist to discuss plans for treatment. I had many questions before proceeding with the treatments, and my husband was unable to be with me for this particular appointment, so I brought a friend with me. Doctors seem to treat you differently when you have your spouse or a friend with you. There is an accountability factor involved when a witness is present, especially if that person is taking notes! The friend that I brought with me took notes of everything that was discussed, typed them up and gave them to me by the next morning. This was extremely helpful, so that my husband and I could discuss our options.

God's hand is in every situation

My husband and I have peace and confidence in knowing that we have a Sovereign God who is in control of every situation. He knew the timing of the diagnosis, so I don't need to question "if only this had been caught eight months earlier." God has placed my husband as my head and so, when he felt strongly that, after praying about various methods of treatment, the Lord was leading in a particular treatment plan, I was able to rest in this, knowing that God was leading us through my husband. God had His hand in every aspect of this entire situation. He has placed many people in my life that I would not have known if this situation had not occurred. He has given my husband and me opportunities to share our faith in God and His mercies, and to be witnesses in proclaiming that His grace truly is sufficient. I am thankful for what God has taught me through having cancer, and I am a step closer in the awareness of my total dependence in Him.

Doctors are not God. Our confidence can **not** be based entirely on their knowledge. They are tools used by God, who can be of great help to us, but they will make mistakes. Unfortunately, our society has become so lawsuit happy that I believe it can affect our receiving proper treatment. Most M.D.s are afraid to admit a mistake, or even ask for forgiveness, in fear of a lawsuit. How sad for them, especially for Christian doctors.

In spite of this, we must remember that we have a Sovereign God who is in control of all situations. We need to take charge of our own healthcare, become informed, and research methods of treatment, including proper nutrition, in assisting our bodies to heal from disease, seeking knowledge from healthcare professionals and, most importantly, seeking God's plan. We need to be ready to forgive when a mistake has occurred, for God is in control of this, too. When we have this proper understanding, fear is taken away, and we are able to rest in Him. Ultimately, our health rests in God's hands.

Part Six:
Infections

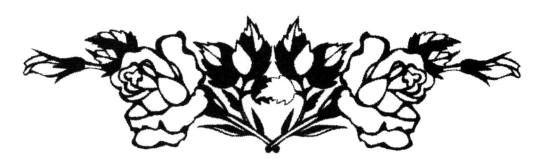

CHAPTER 1
URINARY TRACT INFECTIONS

The most common urinary tract infection is cystitis, an infection of the bladder. Symptoms include: urinary frequency, painful urination with burning, and a sense of urgency with only drops coming out each time. For a variety of reasons, we women are much more likely to have UTIs than men:

- a woman's urethra is closer to the anus;
- sexual intercourse can deposit bacteria near the urethra;
- improper wiping after a bowel movement deposits bacteria near the urethra as well as the vaginal opening;
- feminine hygiene sprays, douches and bubble baths all irritate the normal cleansing process of our bodies;
- underpants made of synthetic material provide an ideal breeding ground for bacteria;
- we may not drink enough, particularly fresh water, to supply the urinary tract with a constant supply of urine to flush it out.

Lifestyle/Dietary Recommendations:

1. Wipe from front to back after bowel movements.
2. Urinate after sexual relations, and practice good hygiene (washing up) afterwards.
3. Avoid feminine hygiene sprays, douches and bubble baths. Douches should not be used during pregnancy except under the advice and direction of a professional healthcare advisor.

4. Wear loose clothing and plain (or pretty) breathable cotton underwear.

5. Drink 2 quarts of pure water daily. Add lemon to increase urine acidity. Urinate often— whenever you feel the need. Do not hold urine while finishing a task—urinate, then come back to whatever you were doing.

6. If urinary symptoms persist with a negative urinalysis, suspect a yeast infection (Part Six, Chapter 2: Vaginal Infections).

7. If your husband is having symptoms too, suggest he follow the supplement guidelines below.

8. If symptoms persist and yeast is not the culprit, investigate the possibility of allergies. My daughter, who is allergic to many foods, has problems with recurrent UTIs.

Nutritional Supplement Recommendations:

1. Cranberry juice concentrate: 1 capsule, 3 times daily taken with 8 ounces of purified water.[1][2]

2. Buffered vitamin C or Ester-C: 500-1,000 mg every 4 hours until the infection has cleared. Maintenance dose: 1,000-1,500 mg daily.

3. Uva ursi, grindelia, pipsissewa, and couchgrass are all herbs that research has shown to be beneficial to the urinary system, especially in the treatment of cystitis.[3] Uva ursi should not be used in large amounts during pregnancy, due to its uterine stimulant properties. Uva ursi's active constituent is arbutin. In the alkaline environment of urine, arbutin is converted into hydroquinone, which kills bacteria. Dosage: 3-5 ml, 3 times daily of a standardized extract, or in capsule or tablet form containing 250 mg of arbutin, 3 times daily.

4. Goldenseal contains berberine, an alkaloid that may prevent UTIs by inhibiting bacteria from adhering to the wall of the urinary bladder.[4]

5. Cornsilk is a demulcent herb (soothing to mucus membranes) that provides relief from the burning of infected urine.

CHAPTER 2
VAGINAL INFECTIONS

The most common vaginal infections are: yeast (Candida albicans), bacterial vaginitis (Bacteriosis vaginosis, often caused by Gardnerella), and Trichomonas (Trichomonas vaginalis). As always, prevention is the best course of action, and so I have given the lifestyle and dietary recommendations first. They are the same for all types of vaginal infections.

Lifestyle and dietary recommendations:

1. Wear cotton underpants.
2. Eliminate or decrease sugar and refined carbohydrate consumption.
3. Use perfume/dye-FREE toilet paper and laundry detergent.
4. Use no feminine hygiene products such as sprays, powders, etc. Daily bathing is sufficient.
5. Clean hands and body before and after intimate relations with your husband (this implies relations only with husband: chastity is necessary for the avoidance of some vaginal infections, which are sexually transmitted).
6. Eat one cup of plain yogurt with live cultures daily.
7. Eat plenty of garlic and make sure the mainstay of your diet is complex carbohydrates and fiber from vegetables, fruits and legumes.

Yeast (Candida Albicans)

Yeast infections are the most common reason that women seek out professional medical attention. The symptoms necessitate some action: genital itching, dryness, inflammation, and heavy, thick white discharge with yeasty-smelling cottage cheese-like clumps. Antibiotic therapy commonly results in yeast infections in women as an undesirable aftereffect. The cause is a fungus called Candida albicans. Candida infections can occur in areas of the body other than the vagina, and can become systemic, where the infection affects the whole body. Many nutritional therapies involve restrictive diets, bowel cleanses, and other life-altering measures. I believe an abrupt change of diet and lifestyle is stressful in itself, and not conducive to getting rid of the "fungus among us." Instead, I have provided some basic recommendations that do not require sweeping, abrupt changes in lifestyle.

Nutritional supplement recommendations:

1. Microwave underpants[1].
2. Place pure acidophilus capsules high in the vagina at bedtime. *Be careful when placing these capsules, or anything else, into the vagina, not to push them into the opening of the cervix.
3. An acidophilus powder or cranberry concentrate powder (1 tablespoon to 1 quart of water) as a douche may be helpful. Douching during pregnancy is a definite risk to both mother and baby. Douching should only be done during pregnancy under the care and instruction of a professional health care provider.
4. A woman may choose to use a clove of garlic (without damaging the clove, or it will be very irritating to vaginal tissue), inserted into her vagina overnight. Some women find this to burn too much. You can check and see. If burning occurs, make up some chamomile tea quickly and douche with the tea, or soak in a tub with lavender, calendula and/or chamomile, allowing the water to enter the vagina to soothe the inflamed tissue.
5. Take ½ teaspoon acidophilus powder with ½ teaspoon Inner Strength™ (EN). Combine with warm water and drink 4-6 times daily during the infection, to re-supply your body with "friendly" bacteria.
6. Swab tea tree oil mixture around the vagina, using gauze soaked in: 1 cup water with 3 drops of tea tree oil. Or use a tea tree oil suppository once daily for 7-10 days[2]. Some women may experience a burning sensation vaginally with intra-vaginal use of tea tree. Proceed with caution. Do not use undiluted tea tree oil. This will burn and cause tissue swelling—my experience speaking!
7. Echinacea may be taken orally. Initial dose: 1,000 mg or 2 mg tincture/tinctract; then 500-1,000 mg every 2-3 hours for 2 days; then three times daily for 3 days; finally twice daily for 5 more days.

8. Pau D'Arco: 500-1,000 mg twice daily for 2-3 weeks. Use with caution during pregnancy.
9. Grapefruit seed extract: 130 mg, twice daily, with plenty of water. This option, as well as number 8 above, are short-term therapies: 2-3 weeks maximum[3].
10. A product by Nutrition Now called Yeast Defense was very helpful for me during a pregnancy in which I had to take antibiotics for a terrible sinus infection. Try 2 capsules of Yeast Defense plus one tablet of garlic every 3 hours, and 1 tablet of pure grapefruit seed extract 3-4 times daily, continuing the therapy for at least 10-14 days.

Bacterial Vaginitis (Bacteriosis vaginosis; Gardnerella)

Symptoms may include: itchy, inflamed vagina with a white or yellowish, thin, highly odorous (fish odor) discharge that may be blood streaked. Frequent, painful urination, cramps or lower back pain may also be present. The husband of an infected woman must be treated too.

Nutritional Supplement Recommendations:

1. Echinacea: 1,000 mg, 4 times daily, or ½ teaspoon Echinacea tincture or tinctract.
2. An echinacea infusion (1 ounce to 2 cups boiling water, steep 10 hours) may be used for douching: 3 tablespoons infusion to 1 quart water. Douche daily for 7 days. You may also douche with bayberry bark. Douching during pregnancy is a risk for both mother and baby, and should only be done under the care and direction of a professional healthcare provider.

Trichomonas (Trichomonas vaginalis)

Symptoms include: itching and inflammation of vulva and vagina, and a prurient greenish-yellow discharge that is slimy or foamy. Anal sexual contact is a major cause of "Trich" because it normally resides in the rectum. Trich is thought only to be passed through sexual contact, although it is conceivable that a woman could wipe from back to front (a real "no-no") and pass the bacteria into her vagina. Men may harbor the organism in their penis without symptoms. It is imperative that both husband and wife be treated. Since Trich cannot live in an acidic environment, the goal in treating an infected woman is to acidify the vagina.

Nutritional Supplement Recommendations:

1. For the husband: 1-2 teaspoons Goldenseal/Myrrh tincture or tinctract, 3 times daily for 10 days; he should also use a Pau D'Arco sitz bath to wash his penis: make a strong infusion of Pau D'Arco (taheebo or lapacho). Soak the penis for 15 minutes, twice daily.

The infusion is made by steeping ½ ounce of Pau D'Arco in 2 cups of water for 20 minutes.

2. A woman can take 2 tablespoons of apple cider vinegar or lemon juice in water twice daily plus 5,000 mg vitamin C.

3. A douche of: 2 tablespoons white vinegar and 1 tablespoon activated charcoal powder to 1 quart of water may be used daily for 1 week, then every other day for the following week, and then twice weekly for 2 more weeks.

4. Garlic cloves (as described for yeast) may be used every 3 hours for 3 days, then once a day, overnight, for 4 more days. The third week, garlic suppositories or capsules may be used every other day, then twice in the fourth week.[4]

5. In one study, Pau D'Arco (lapacho) extract was applied in the vagina using gauze soaked in the extract. A fresh-soaked gauze was renewed every 24 hours. The treatment was highly effective.[5]

6. A lactobacillus vaccine called Solcotrichovac was used in a study of 444 women, which yielded a 92.5% cure rate after one vaccination of the inactivated microorganisms.[6]

7. Bee propolis extract has been shown to have lethal effects on Trich in vitro.[7]

CHAPTER 3
CHLAMYDIA AND HERPES

These two sexually-transmitted diseases differ from those we have looked at in their severity, and in their long-term effects on both women and their unborn children.

Chlamydia

Chlamydia is a very common bacterial sexually-transmitted disease in the United States. It has been called the "silent disease" because often there are no symptoms at all. Until recently, tests were often unreliable in detecting the bacteria. This has been problematic, because chlamydia is the leading cause of pelvic inflammatory disease (PID). If left untreated, this disease causes 20 to 40% of female infertility, and can be a cause of tubal pregnancy, due to scarring from the prolonged pelvic infection it can cause. When there are symptoms, they usually include inflammation of the urethra and cervix, burning urination, excessive vaginal bleeding, fever (usually mild) and abdominal pain. Symptoms may begin two to three weeks after the infection. Pregnant women are tested for chlamydia, because it can be passed to their baby during a vaginal birth, leading to pneumonia, eye infection and blindness.

Doctors generally treat chlamydia with doxycycline for seven to ten days, as well as prescribing other antibiotics as needed. Natural treatments are not offered here as an alternative to the standard medical treatment, as we feel that the doxycycline is necessary for preventing severe damage from chlamydia. We will instead be offering adjunct (additional) therapy to enhance the action of the antibiotics, and strengthen the body.

Dietary and Lifestyle Recommendations:

1. Eliminate as much sugar as possible from the diet.
2. Eat at least 5 fruits and vegetables a day. Enjoy whole grains, beans, and legumes, and remember that meat should be a side dish, not the main portion on your plate.
3. Include a probiotic supplement before meals. Purchase a refrigerated probiotic so the good bacteria will definitely be alive and in top form.

Nutritional Supplement Recommendations:

1. Support the immune system with echinacea and garlic. Take standard doses twice daily.
2. Support the liver with herbs such as dandelion or milk thistle.
3. Include a high-quality multivitamin/mineral supplement for women in your daily routine.

Herpes

Herpes Simplex Viruses, both Type I (HSV-I) and Type II (HSV-II) are recurrent viral infections that may remain dormant for short or long periods after the initial, primary infection. They can recur at any time, usually during times of physical or emotional stress.

HSV-I

Type I is the cause of the common fever blister in, on or around the mouth. It may also be found on the fingers of the hand in individuals who touch their fever blisters often.[1] If lesions (fever blisters) are present, oral contact with others should be avoided. Type I may be transmitted to the genitals: ten percent of genital herpes is Type I. Hand washing should be employed often, using warm, soapy water.

HSV-II

Type II herpes is almost always transmitted sexually. Skin-to-skin contact is necessary to contract herpes.[2] The incubation period from exposure is usually six to ten days, and initial symptoms are intense vulvar itching, burning, tingling and tenderness. There are one or many small or large thin-walled, fluid-filled vesicles that may appear over the vulva, vestibule, perianal area, or inner surfaces of the thigh, inside the vagina and/or on the cervix. Urination may be painful because of lesions. Vesicles rupture forming painful ulcers. At this stage, most infected women feel ill and have a low-grade temperature.

Lesions usually regress, with the pain disappearing in two to four weeks. Lesions recur in fifty percent of persons infected with the herpes simplex virus. Recurrences are usually less severe and of shorter duration.[3] Prior to recurring outbreaks, some experience a prodromal phase of tingling, neuralgia, and a sensation of pressure or increased vaginal discharge.[4]

HSV-II may transplacentally infect an unborn baby, and cause congenital defects, although this is rare. Congenital defects most often occur with a primary infection of a pregnant woman. There is an increased risk of miscarriage and prematurity for babies of mothers who are infected during pregnancy.

Babies born to mothers infected at the time of birth have a forty to sixty percent chance of being infected. For this reason, a cesarean is indicated if a woman has a current outbreak when she goes into labor.[5]

Lifestyle and Dietary Recommendations:

1. Avoid foods high in arginine: almonds, brazil nuts, cashews, hazelnuts, peanuts, pecans, walnuts, chocolate, gelatin. Restrict amounts of: coconut, barley, corn, oats, wheat, pasta, brussel sprouts.[6]
2. Do eat foods high in lysine: milk (See discussion on milk in Part 2), soybeans, beef, poultry, sour cream, yogurt, fish, eggs, buckwheat.[7]
3. Icy cloths or ice packs may provide pain relief for lesions.
4. Keep lesions clean and dry; cotton underwear is a must.
5. Wash your hands often, and do not touch or pick at lesions.

Nutritional Supplement Recommendations:

1. L-Lysine is an amino acid that is highly recommended to combat herpes outbreaks: 1,200-3,000 mg of L-Lysine daily.[8]
2. Lactobacillus acidophilus may help relieve symptoms of outbreaks as well as prevent future recurrences: 3 capsules daily, or ¼-½ teaspoon 3 times daily of powder. Only purchase refrigerated probiotic supplements.[9]
3. Herbs exhibiting anti-viral activity in current research against herpes are: Uva ursi[10], 2 capsules three times daily (use caution during pregnancy, as it has uterine-stimulating properties); bilberry[11], 2 capsules 3 times daily; buckthorn[12], 1 capsule 3 times daily (use caution during pregnancy as it has bowel-stimulating properties); echinacea[13], 500 mg every 2-3 hours during an outbreak; red raspberry[14], 2 capsules 3 times daily; blue-green algae[15], 1,000-3,000 mg daily; licorice[16], 2 to 4 capsules daily (use caution during pregnancy due to phytosterols in the plant). Obviously, a woman will not want to use all of these herbs.
4. For herbal topical antiviral herbs, clove oil and tea tree oil have both been found to inhibit the herpes virus.[17]

5. Peppermint has been shown to inhibit and kill the herpes simplex virus, among many other microorganisms.[18]
6. Herpilyn, by Enzymatic Therapy, may be applied topically to lesions for speedier healing.
7. Bee Propolis has been shown in studies to reduce the viral titer of herpes simplex virus and reduce viral synthesis, as well as cut recovery time in half for patients with post-herpetic trophic keratitis and/or post-herpetic nebula.[19] [20]

Can herpes ever be eradicated?

Echinacea root and burdock root, in equal amounts, have been reported to prevent outbreaks and eradicate the herpes virus from the body system if taken for six months: ten days on, ten days off, at a dosage of 500-1,000 mg of each, two to three times daily. I have no clinically documented experience with "eliminating" the herpes virus, but this combination of herbs, at the very least, has proved beneficial in clinical practice in limiting an outbreak and preventing recurrence.

Part Seven:
Menopause

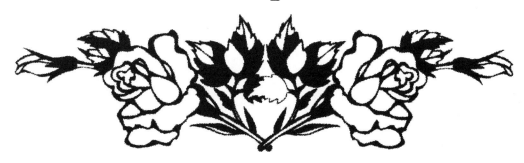

CHAPTER 1
HORMONAL HEALTH

Menopause is commonly referred to as "the change" women go through as they pass from their childbearing years to the years of being, as the scriptures tell us, older women who should teach the younger women how to manage their homes and children. Menopausal symptoms may begin several years prior to the cessation of menses, a time known as perimenopause. The first clue many women have that they are nearing menopause is a change in the regularity of their menstrual cycles, or in the quality of their cycles, which may mean heavier bleeding, and perhaps more pain. A woman is considered post-menopausal when she has not had a period in one to two years.

The average age of menopause for North American women is fifty-one, although there appears to be a trend towards earlier onset. The usual age range is from mid forties to mid fifties, although menopause can occur naturally in women aged thirty-six to sixty. In cultures where women begin bearing children at an early age, they generally come to menopause at around thirty-six. Most of us will notice that we go through menopause at the same time as our mothers and grandmothers did.

The symptoms associated with the approach of menopause include hot flashes, vaginal dryness or itching, incontinence, heavy and irregular periods, and poor concentration and memory. Some women also experience depression, insomnia, fatigue, loss of muscle tone, weight gain, and joint and muscle pain. Some women experience no symptoms at all. Some conditions actually improve with the onset of menopause, due to the diminished production of estrogen: uterine fibroids, breast cysts and endometriosis.

More and more, we are finding that the habits we adopt in our early years of womanhood allow us either to be able to embrace this change in a healthful fashion, or require us to persevere through a fiery trial. For instance, the increased risk of osteoporosis has been thought to be caused by a lack of estrogen; however, new evidence is coming to light that shows it is the amount a girl child's bones are properly calcified prior to the onset of menses that protects her from osteoporosis later in life. Another factor that increases the risk of difficult menopausal years is not properly taking care of oneself during the childbearing years. Women who choose not to let pregnancy slow them down at all, but who bounce back into their normal activities within days of giving birth, appear more likely to suffer the ill effects of menopausal symptoms.

There are natural alternatives to the hormonal-replacement therapy (HRT) prescribed by allopathic and osteopathic physicians. In my opinion, trying the natural alternatives is preferable to going straight to pharmaceuticals due to the fact that HRT carries its own risks and side effects. I have this common scenario: a woman begins HRT, only to have her blood pressure increase. So another medication is prescribed for that, and then the thyroid goes haywire, requiring another—and so forth, until she is a walking pharmacy with her case of pills. We will address natural hormone replacement protocol here, including the attention that has been given in recent years to natural progesterone crèmes.

Dietary and lifestyle recommendations:

1. Mothers, begin now to give your daughters calcium supplements each day prior to the onset of their menses.
2. Take care of yourself during the childbearing years. Slow down and enjoy the baby in your womb. Rejoice in those first few weeks of cuddling your new blessing. All your other activities will be there later.
3. As the menopausal years begin, eat a whole foods diet with an emphasis on soy products, fennel, celery, parsley, nuts and seeds. These contain natural estrogen precursors, and also protect against breast cancer.
4. Avoid a high-fat diet. The Kronenberg survey of 2,000 women showed that women on low-fat diets had fewer symptoms of menopause than others. Low-fat, high-fiber is the way to go during these years.
5. Eat deep-sea fish, which contain omega-3 fatty acids.
6. Eat soy products, if thyroid problems are not an issue.
7. Eat plenty of beans and legumes, which are natural sources of phytoestrogens.
8. Exercise regularly. A Swedish study showed that exercise is beneficial in reducing menopausal symptoms, and it certainly helps to reduce the risk of developing osteoporosis.
9. Frequent sexual relations with your husband help to reduce the incidence of hot flashes, and may help retain vaginal tone and lubrication.

10. Kegel exercises for the PC muscle (the one that allows you to stop the flow of urine) 100 times daily will help to keep internal organs in place and improve vaginal tone.

Nutritional supplement recommendations:

1. Take a flax oil supplement daily: 1-2 tablespoons, or the equivalent amount in capsules. The oil must be kept refrigerated to avoid rancidity.
2. Take a phytoestrogen-rich herb formula such as: Femtrol (Enzymatic Therapy), Change-O-Life (Nature's Way), FemChange (Nature's Herbs) or Men-O-Pause (Liquid Light).
3. Herbs specifically helpful for hot flashes are: angelica or dong quai (Angelica sinensis), licorice root (Glycyrrhiza glabra), chaste berry (Vitex agnus-castus) and black cohosh (Cimicifuga racemosa). The above formulas should contain these herbs, and may be taken at a dosage of 2 capsules 3 times daily.
4. If additional help is needed, gamma-oryzanol (ferulic acid), a growth-promoting substance found in grains and isolated from rice bran oil, may be taken at a dosage of 300 mg daily. Gamma-oryzanol also helps to lower blood cholesterol and triglyceride levels.
5. Take a calcium supplement: 1200 mg daily, and a magnesium supplement: 600 mg daily.
6. Take vitamin C: 2-3 g daily, and vitamin E: 800 IU daily, with meals.

Shonda's favorite menopause supplement protocol:

❀ Equilibrium by NF Formulas: take as directed on bottle.
❀ Remifemin by Enzymatic Therapy: take as directed on the package. If depression is a problem, use the version with St. John's Wort.
❀ Calcium with isoflavone: take 1,000 mg daily.
❀ Evening Primrose Oil or Flaxseed oil: take 1 tablespoon 2-3 times daily.

I have found this combination of supplements to be highly effective. If they don't work for you, try some of the others above.

Chapter 2
Cardiovascular Disease

Current conventional medical thought is that a woman's risk of developing heart disease increases as her estrogen levels decrease through menopause. Women who are post-menopausal need to lower fat intake, and incorporate exercise into a daily regimen, so that the risk of cardiovascular disease does not increase to match that of middle-aged men. At menopause, because of naturally lower estrogen levels, a woman's risk of cardiovascular disease triples.

As women, we often don't think that we are at great risk of developing cardiovascular disease, but it is the overall leading cause of death in women, killing two hundred and fifty thousand American women each year. Most studies on heart disease are done on men, but that may change in the near future, as we realize that women who develop coronary artery disease are more likely to die from it, or suffer from a major reduction in quality of life, than their male counterparts.

Many cardiologists are beginning to be more aggressive about treating women who complain of chest pain. My own family history meant that, last year, I required a cardiovascular workup. I was experiencing some chest pains, and as I have a maternal history that is quite significant for heart disease, the cardiologist took me through all the hoops to make certain I was not developing heart problems. As it turned out, I was not. The chest pains were probably caused by stress. However, he insisted that he continue to monitor my cardio health every six months, due to my family history. Although I did not enjoy all the tests, none were invasive, and I was glad that he took this approach.

Several Conditions May be Involved in Cardiovascular Disease:

High blood pressure:

Also known as hypertension, high blood pressure is the most common chronic medical condition. It affects seventeen to twenty-five million women, and is more common in post-menopausal women than it is in men. Normal blood pressure fluctuates throughout the day, depending on our physical exertions and our emotional state. The risk is from continuously high blood pressure, which can damage arterial walls.

Recent (1989) research at the University of Cambridge, England, helps us to understand and evaluate this risk. Normal, healthy women had their blood pressure monitored throughout the day. Dr. Kevin Dalton, who conducted this study, found that their systolic pressure fluctuated up to forty points; their diastolic readings fluctuated as much as twenty points. The average fluctuation was between twenty and thirty millimeters of mercury within a ten minute period.[1] It is important to view these normal fluctuations as just that—normal. A woman with consistently high blood pressure, or significantly rising blood pressure, should take measures to help bring it back to normal.

Values that are considered high blood pressure in adults are:
- ❀ Borderline: 120-160/90-94
- ❀ Mild: 140-160/95-104
- ❀ Moderate: 140-180/105-114
- ❀ Severe: 160+/115+.

A common reading for an adult is 120(Systolic)/80(Diastolic). In adults, prescription drugs do not seem to be the answer for those in the borderline to moderate range. In fact, these drugs often produce unnecessary side effects that increase the risk for heart disease. Two definitive trials, the Australian and Medical Research Council trials, as well as five other large trials, including the famous Multiple Risk Factor Intervention Trial (MRFIT), compared patients receiving drug treatment with those receiving a placebo, i.e. no actual treatment. These studies have shown that the drugs offer no benefit in protecting against heart disease in borderline to moderate hypertension.[2] In fact, the American Journal of Cardiology published an article in which the following quotation was found: Few patients with uncomplicated marginal hypertension require drug treatment. . .there is little evidence these patients (with marginal hypertension) will achieve enough benefit to justify the costs and adverse effects of anti-hypertension drug treatment.[3]

Yearly sales of blood pressure medications are estimated to be greater than ten billion dollars. Eighty percent of patients are in the mild to moderate range; if they no longer were prescribed these medications, this could result in an eight billion dollar yearly loss to drug companies. Doctors who prescribe this treatment might also feel the pinch in their pockets. A Journal of the American Medical Association article stated: treatment of hypertension has become the leading reason for visits to physicians as well as for drug prescriptions.[4] Yet, natural alternatives to treatment for mild to moderate hypertension, if employed, would obviously lend substantial benefit.

Cardiac arrhythmia:

This rather frightening term means an irregular heartbeat. Sometimes, the heart may seem to skip a beat, then pound harder to catch up: this is an arrhythmia, although it may be perfectly normal. Heart palpitations fit into this category. They are usually harmless, and may be caused by overexertion, anemia, or may happen during panic attacks or hot flashes. Severe arrhythmias may result in dizziness, a cold sweat and shortness of breath. If you experience any persistently irregular heartbeat, you should discuss it with a physician.

Heart valve disease:

Our hearts have four chambers, each with a valve that opens as the heart pumps, and closes as it rests. This keeps the blood flowing in the right direction, without "backwashing." Symptoms of improper functioning of one or more of these valves include: palpitations, chest pain, fatigue, breathlessness, even fainting. Mitral valve prolapse is a relatively common example, affecting five percent of all women. Although rarely dangerous, it can cause worrisome chest pain. Caffeine seems to be a major aggravator of this condition. Certain types of mitral valve prolapse sometime become serious enough to warrant surgery.

Angina and coronary artery disease:

Angina refers to chest pain that occurs behind the breastbone. Angina attacks occur when a greater demand is placed on the heart, but the heart is unable to get enough oxygen to perform the task. This may mean that the arteries carrying blood to the heart have been narrowed by plaque accumulation, a condition called coronary artery disease, or atherosclerosis. The attacks may only last a few minutes; but, when they occur often and without stimulus, there is more likelihood of a heart attack occurring.

Heart attack:

Medical personnel refer to a heart attack as a "MI", which is short for the technical term "myocardial infarction" or "myocardial infarct." A heart attack occurs because the heart does not receive enough oxygen and nutrients to function, so parts of the heart muscle begin to die. This usually occurs due to blockage of blood flow by fatty plaque, blood clots, or a combination of both. A mild heart attack can be silent: you may not even know you have had one, or it may be mistaken for indigestion. However, common symptoms are: pain that radiates from the chest to the left arm or the neck, jaw or back, sweating, nausea, and/or fainting. A heart attack can be diagnosed by heart scans or by blood analysis.

Congestive heart failure:

Congestive heart failure results when a damaged or weakened heart cannot pump enough blood to keep the body healthy. Symptoms include: difficulty breathing, fatigue, and fluid retention, especially in the lungs. The most common causes of congestive heart failure are: chronic high blood pressure, a previous heart attack, heart valve disorders, coronary artery disease, or a combination of these factors.

Stroke:

A stroke occurs when a blood vessel in the brain becomes blocked or bursts, damaging the brain because of lack of oxygen to that area. This usually occurs because of the narrowing (hardening) of blood vessels, or blockage of a vessel by a blood clot, which blocks blood flow to the brain. The result can be paralysis, loss of brain function, or death. Full-mouth dental x-rays are being simultaneously used now to ascertain the health of blood vessels leading to the brain, as some blockages may be seen on these x-rays.

Health Care Recommendations for Cardiovascular Fitness:

High blood pressure:

Lifestyle and dietary recommendations:

1. Reduce or eliminate high-risk lifestyle factors: caffeine and alcohol intake, lack of exercise, stress and smoking. Coffee consumption: blood pressure rises with five or more cups of

coffee per day. Alcohol intake should not exceed one ounce of alcohol daily (this means 2 oz. of liquor, 4 oz. of wine, or 12 oz. of beer) for those with high blood pressure.

2. Eliminate high-risk dietary factors, which include: obesity, too much sodium, not enough potassium, a low fiber, high-sugar diet, a diet high in saturated fat and low essential fatty acids, and a diet low in calcium, magnesium and vitamin C.

3. Increase potassium intake. Sodium restriction is not advised; it is the potassium to sodium intake ratio that is important. Researchers recommend a potassium to sodium ratio of 5:1 for maintaining good health. The average American diet has a ratio of 1:2. The benefit of added potassium really needs to come from the diet—not from drugs or supplements.

4. Increase plant food consumption. Vegetarians generally have lower blood pressure levels, and a correspondingly lower incidence of consistent high blood pressure and cardiovascular disease.

5. Restrict intake of sucrose (table sugar), which elevates blood pressure, probably because of the increased adrenaline production resulting in increased blood vessel constriction and increased sodium retention. On the other hand, foods containing complex carbohydrates, that are high in fiber, lower blood pressure.

6. Omega-3 fatty acids lower cholesterol as well as decreasing blood pressure. Double-blind studies demonstrate that fish oil (EPA or eicosapentaenoic acid) supplements, or linolenic acid from flaxseed oil, are effective for lowering blood pressure.[5] The recommended intake is 1 tablespoon of flaxseed oil per day, either as cold-processed oil used in salad dressings, or in supplemental form.

7. Studies have shown several special foods to be particularly helpful in lowering blood pressure: celery: 4 ribs per day; garlic: 3 or more cloves per day, and onions; nuts and seeds, or their oils, for their EFA (essential fatty acid) content; coldwater fish; green, leafy vegetables (a rich source of calcium and/or magnesium); whole grains and legumes for fiber; and foods rich in vitamin C, such as broccoli, green peppers, and citrus fruits.

8. Relax and pray.

9. Exercise regularly.

Nutritional supplements:

1. Calcium: 1000-1500 mg daily; magnesium 500-1000 mg daily. The highly absorbable forms are citrate, orotates, aspartates, or Krebs-cycle chelate intermediates.

2. Ginkgo and hawthorn combination of herbs: 2 in the morning, 2 before bedtime. Generally this supplement must be taken 2 weeks before an observable lowering of blood pressure.[6]

3. Coenzyme Q10: 20 mg, 3 times daily.

4. Garlic: 600-900 mg daily. Study has shown this level of supplement to lower blood pressure.[7]

Atherosclerosis (Coronary artery disease):

1. Dietary and lifestyle recommendations: Reduce serum cholesterol levels by consuming a wide variety of whole foods, concentrating on a diet rich in vegetables and fruits.
2. Get regular physical exercise.
3. Cease cigarette smoking.
4. Limit coffee consumption to less than 6 cups daily. Tea consumption does not appear to be a problem.
5. Eliminate alcohol consumption, as this leads to an increase in serum cholesterol triglycerides and uric acid levels, as well as to high blood pressure.
6. Increase dietary fiber intake, especially the gel-forming or mucilaginous fibers (flaxseed, oat bran, pectin, etc), cold-pressed oils and fish.
7. Ginger, garlic and onions should be used liberally in foods.
8. Limit refined sugar consumption.

Nutritional supplements:

1. Begin a supplementation program with a high quality multi-vitamin and mineral daily supplement.
2. Take garlic supplements. A recent, 4-year, double-blind, controlled study on the effect of garlic on people with atherosclerosis showed that the participants who took garlic each day experienced a reduction in arterial plaque over the 4-year period. Those not taking garlic experienced a marked increase in their plaque levels. Garlic supplementation is definitely indicated.
3. Vitamin C: a total of at least 2,000 mg daily.
4. Vitamin E: at least 200 IU daily.
5. A fiber supplement of psyllium seed, guar gum, or other water-soluble fiber: 5,000 mg (5 grams) daily.
6. Flaxseed oil: 1-2 tablespoons daily.
7. Omega EPA oils: 5-10 g daily.
8. Carnitine: 900 mg daily. Carnitine has been shown to be effective therapeutically in the treatment of atherosclerotic heart disease. Heart function depends on an adequate carnitine supply. Carnitine also increases HDL levels, while decreasing triglyceride and cholesterol levels.[8]
9. Bromelain: 300-500 mg, 3 times daily at least 30 minutes before meals. Bromelain is the proteolytic enzyme found in pineapples. It has been shown to inhibit platelet aggregation, improve angina pain, reduce blood pressure, and break down atherosclerotic plaques.

10. Mesoglycan: 100 mg daily. This supplement improves the structure, function and integrity of the arteries.[9]
11. Ginkgo biloba capsules: twice daily, in the morning and 30 minutes before bedtime, to improve blood flow.

High Cholesterol and Triglyceride Levels:

Cholesterol, carried in blood plasma by lipoproteins, is certainly a buzz word these days. Cholesterol is often referred to as "good" or "bad." The "good" cholesterol is the high-density lipoprotein (HDL). HDL transports cholesterol to the liver for metabolism and excretion, and protects against heart disease. Low-density lipoprotein (LDL) transports cholesterol to tissue. This is the "bad" cholesterol that increases a person's risk of heart disease. The table below shows recommended values for cholesterol levels.

TYPE	NORMAL LEVELS
Total Cholesterol	less than 200mg/dl
LDL	less than 130mg/dl
HDL	greater than 35 mg/dl
Triglycerides	50-150 mg/dl

Sources: Murray, Michael T., N.D. The Healing Power of Foods. Rocklin, CA: Prima Publishing, 1993.

Lifestyle and dietary recommendations:

1. Reduce saturated fats (milk and other animal fats) in the diet. Saturated fats prompt the liver (which manufactures the majority of cholesterol in the body) to produce more cholesterol. Unsaturated fats tell the liver to produce less.
2. Remember that not all fats are bad. In fact, essential fatty acids (EFAs) are great. These EFAs are found in marine fish oils (Omega-3), cold-pressed safflower, sunflower, canola, Evening Primrose, black currant and borage oils. These EFAs actually provide the building blocks for the chemical regulators known as prostaglandins.

3. Eat nuts and seeds. They do have a high oil content; however, a study of 26,473 Americans found that those who consumed the most nuts were the least obese. This study also demonstrated that higher nut consumption was associated with protective effects against heart attacks.[10] Nuts are best purchased in shells free from splits, cracks, stains, holes or other surface problems. They should be stored in a cool, dry environment. Hulled nuts and seeds should be stored in airtight containers in the refrigerator or freezer.

4. Eliminate margarine. Butter may be used in limited quantities. Canola and olive oils should be used for cooking.

5. Eat a whole foods diet. This is essential for lowering cholesterol levels. A whole food diet is high in fruits, vegetables, whole grains and legumes, and naturally high-fiber. Fiber absorbs bile, which contains cholesterol, and moves it along the intestines for excretion. Lack of fiber means the bile and cholesterol are reabsorbed.

Nutritional supplements:

1. Gugulipid, from guggal or mukul myrrh tree: extracts standardized to contain 25mg of gugulipid per tablet, taken 3 times daily, have been shown in clinical studies to be effective in lowering cholesterol or triglyceride levels.[11][12]

2. Garlic and onions: numerous studies have shown that these lower LDL cholesterol and triglycerides, while raising HDL cholesterol. The equivalent of 1 clove of garlic and/or half an onion per day is necessary to give a 10 to 15% reduction in total cholesterol.[13][14][15]

3. Pantethene: 900 mg daily is the standard dosage for efficacy. Pantethene is the active form of pantothenic acid. It has been evaluated for effectiveness in lowering cholesterol and triglycerides. However, it is a fairly expensive nutritional supplement, which should be saved for elevated triglyceride levels.[16][17]

4. Other nutrients recommended for elevated cholesterol and triglyceride levels are chromium and vitamin C.[18]

CHAPTER 3
OSTEOPOROSIS

Osteoporosis refers to a condition where the bones are no longer solidly calcified. Instead, they have become brittle, easy to break. Osteoporosis is most common in post-menopausal white and Oriental women. Many older women with brittle bones express their fear of falling and breaking a hip, an all-too-common experience that can considerably reduce the length and quality of life.

A woman's bones begin to lose mass after age thirty-five. This loss reaches a peak in the first five to nine years after menopause. Early intervention measures to build our bones and protect them from this loss is vital to our overall health.

In the early part of this book, we talked about the benefit of breastfeeding on preventing osteoporosis in our daughters, as well as the benefit of providing them with plenty of calcium before they begin menstruating to reduce their risk. But what can we do, in our middles ages and beyond, to protect our bones?

Dietary and Lifestyle Recommendations:

1. Exercise now to prevent problems later. Women who exercise regularly retain more bone mass than those who are more sedentary. Get off that couch and get walking!
2. Consider weight-lifting. Women can increase their bone density by lifting weights at least twice weekly. If you can't get to a gym to lift weights, make those cans of beans work for you in many ways!

3. Eat a diet full with the variety of God's provision for us: fruits, vegetables, whole grains, nuts, seeds, beans, legumes. Limit meat consumption: excess protein (more than 70 grams daily) can cause loss of calcium through the kidneys. It also causes strain on the kidneys.

4. If you can't drink milk (buy the organic brand), eat plenty of salmon, figs, and green, leafy vegetables. Don't forget those wonderful mustard, turnip, and radish greens, and the collards, too. Drink lemon water while you munch away; that boosts the assimilation of the nutrients.

5. Eat soy products for their phytoestrogens, which help protect from osteoporosis. Only half a cup of tofu every day can make a big difference.

6. Avoid excessive alcohol, caffeine, sodium and phosphoric acid intake. Soda pops are a particular problem, as they may contain both caffeine and phosphoric acid.

Nutritional Supplements:

1. Calcium citrate with isoflavones: 1,500 mg daily, added to the calcium supplement.

2. Vitamin D: 700 IU daily, increases calcium absorption, particularly during the winter months when there is not much sunlight.

3. Magnesium: 250-750 mg daily. For optimum nutrient balance, I prefer to take half my magnesium dosage in my calcium supplement. Magnesium has been shown to arrest bone loss, or increase bone density, in people with osteoporosis.

4. A multi-vitamin with these nutrients: zinc, copper, boron, manganese, silicon, "stable strontium," folic acid, B-vitamins, and vitamin K.

5. Horsetail: this provides a rich source of silicon that is needed for osteoporosis.

6. The recommendations for hormonal support for the post-menopausal woman should be followed.

7. I like a daily tea of nettles, oatstraw and red raspberry, to provide a natural source of calcium, magnesium, and silica. It tastes wonderful. Steep 4 tablespoons of the herb in 1 quart of water. Sweeten with frozen apple juice concentrate, and squeeze in a quarter lemon, to aid assimilation of the nutrients and give it a bit of a tang.

Part Eight:
Weight Loss

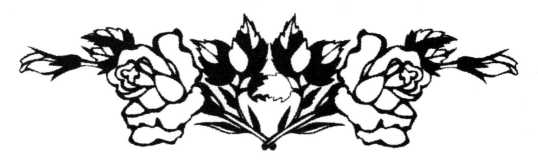

While chatting with one of the women from my church this morning, we were laughing about the change that occurs in a woman's body past a "certain age:" a little extra padding on the rib cage, widening "seat" and for those women who've borne children, looking down one day to find that the skin that once was so taut and firm over the lower abdomen actually has an overhang. Some of this padding is a normal part, perhaps even beneficial part, of growing older. Fat cells store estrogen, so a little extra padding can help some women get over the "hump" of reduced estrogen production by using up the estrogen in their fat cells (if they are diligent to exercise, and thus release that stored estrogen).

Some women struggle with excess weight gain beginning in their thirties and forties; others experience a challenge their entire lives because they add on pounds too easily. Whatever the cause, the onset of middle age spread, or just a lifetime of extra padding, we only have to look in bookstores, health food stores and even department stores to find the latest diet books promising quick weight loss that can be maintained over the long-term.

If there is one area of health and nutrition that disappoints me, it is the ability of nearly anyone to cook up a diet, base it on questionable science, and promote it as the way to "eat your way to skinny" or "starve your way to skinny." Skinny, without real health, is not much better than chubby without health. The question is what we are really looking for in our quest for the right size.

Not so long ago, I couldn't gain weight for the health of me. I was so thin that I was constantly being questioned as to whether I had anorexia. I was not very healthy, nor did I really look healthy—I looked like emaciated. In the past few years, I suddenly experienced a weight gain of about twenty pounds, which placed me, finally, within my normal weight limits. This was a great place to be. With my recent pregnancy, I started out at the upper end of my normal weight chart and still gained my normal thirty-five to forty pounds in pregnancy. This has placed me at a higher weight that I have ever been at before. While birthing a child is a very quick weight-loss program, I will still have a ways to go, over the next year or so, before I will be at my pre-pregnancy weight. I am older now. My body no longer looks like that of a twenty-year-old, and it no longer bounces back the way it did when I was younger. I have traded the "Twiggy" look for more of a "Renaissance-woman" look.

I am not discouraged, though, because I have seen over and over that a well-balanced whole foods diet, combined with regular exercise, is the key to long-term weight loss, weight maintenance and overall body health. The suggestions you will read here are not a promise of quick weight loss, although that could happen. The recommendations will not necessarily make you look like a starlet. These dietary guidelines will not cater to desires to eat only your favorite foods, or desires to not have to give up foods you enjoy but that put on the pounds.

The limited calorie, whole foods diet, combined with the exercise program you will see on these pages will grant weight loss over time, increase your energy, boost your immune system and resistance to chronic disease, as well as give a strong foundation for complete health. You can stuff a dishcloth in your kitchen drain in lieu of a real drain stopper, but it won't work for long. The water will still slowly leak out and you will be refilling the sink over and over again. Invest in a drain stopper, and the water will remain until you decide to drain it. Quick fixes don't generally work for the long-term; they are temporary. What I propose for us is long-term health gain with sensible weight loss!

Lifestyle and Dietary Recommendations:

1. Decrease calories and add exercise. Caloric intake should not go below 1,200 calories daily. One can "afford" 1,500 to 2,000 calories if the amount of exercise is increased. I find it best to decrease caloric intake over a period of weeks, rather than making an abrupt change, unless you are simply ready and willing for lots of denial. The more successful programs allow at least six weeks for a person to decrease calories and become used to smaller portions. Exercise should be slowly added to the daily or weekly routine, as too much in the beginning can be stressful to body muscles, including the heart.

2. There is no "miracle diet." The key to overcoming the set point of fat cells appears to be increasing the fat cells' exposure to insulin. This does not mean eat all protein or limit all fat. It means that we must be controlled in our eating, consuming the highest quality foods in smaller quantities than we may desire, and eating only small amounts of natural fats: olive oil, nuts, seeds, small amounts of real butter.

3. Eat more high-nutrient foods. If the body feels starved, metabolism will slow down and less fat will be burned. Whole grains, beans and legumes, nuts and seeds, as well as vegetables, provide high-nutrient value as well as fiber and protein, which cut down on the amount of food eaten. The daily required amount of protein from meat—or this can be from a vegetarian source, if desired—is about the size of a deck of playing cards.

4. Snacking should be avoided unless it is with foods that expend the same amount of calories to eat as they contain. Vegetables that contain a high amount of water are good for snacks: celery, alfalfa sprouts, bell peppers, bok choy, cabbage, chicory, cucumber, Chinese cabbage, endive, escarole, lettuce, parsley, radishes, spinach, turnips and watercress, to name just a few. You won't gain extra calories and weight from these foods.

5. Exercise should be fifteen to twenty minutes of aerobic activity, three to four times weekly. Walking is an excellent form of exercise for women. Walking is low-impact aerobic exercise that won't harm the joints over the long-term. For regular exercise information, Naturally Healthy Living magazine has a regular column, "Fit and Trim," that gives guidelines for women on how to lose weight and gain good muscle tone, without having to devote our entire lives to exercise.

Nutritional Supplement Recommendations:

1. Fiber supplements seem to be beneficial, through providing bulk in the stomach which decreases food requirements. Supplementation may come from psyllium, guar gum, glucomannan, or pectin: up to 5 grams daily. This should not be necessary for those consuming adequate amounts of fiber in their daily meals. Any fiber supplements must always be taken with a full, 8-ounce glass of water, so as not to cause constipation.

2. Michael T. Murray, N.D., in his excellent book Natural Alternatives to Over-the-Counter and Prescription Drugs,[1] recommends thermogenic herb formulas for weight-loss. The thermogenic formulas work by activating the sympathetic nervous system, which increases metabolism and thermogenesis. Moms who are still breastfeeding need to be cautious because of the stimulant activity of these herbs. If her baby responds to the herbs passed through the breast milk, a nursing mother should discontinue the thermogenic formula immediately. Herbal combinations with synergistic (combining two or more substances to create a stronger action) effects: ephedra (ma huang) is amplified by green tea (Camellia sinesis) or cola nut (Cola nitida) and coffee or black tea. Ephedrine from the Ephedra plant (ma huang) promotes weight loss in experimental and clinical studies by increasing the metabolic rate of fat tissue and decreasing appetite. Ephedrine's action is greatly enhanced by caffeine. 30 mg of ephedrine to 100 mg caffeine is Murray's recommended dosage. This should be taken early in the day and all other stimulants should be eliminated. Thermogenic formulas should not be used in people with high blood pressure, heart disease, or those on antidepressants, without consulting their physician. There have been cases of young women using ephedrine in very large doses with fatal effects. For those interested in using thermogenic formulas, I strongly recommend the purchase of Dr. Murray's book.

3. For appetite control, a special form of the amino acid tryptophan, known in health food circles as 5-hydroxytryptophan or 5-HTP, is a new approach used in weight loss. This type of tryptophan is not the type that caused illness in folks several years ago, due to a contaminated batch from Japan. 5-HTP is the middle step of the process in which the body transforms tryptophan into the brain chemical, serotonin. Serotonin levels are low in many people, as a consequence of high-stress lifestyles. People who have benefited from using 5-HTP to raise serotonin levels in the body include those who: are overweight, crave sugar and other simple carbohydrates, experience bouts of depression, get frequent headaches, and have vague muscle aches and pains. Normal serotonin levels help ensure that the switch in our digestive tract that signals the brain to tell us when we have had enough food, works properly. Dosages for 5-HTP range from 50 mg three times daily, taken twenty minutes before meals, up to 300 mg three times daily. Start off with perhaps a 100 mg dosage for one month, and increase the dosage only if no result is seen, to 200 mg for a month, then up to 300 mg for a month after that. Do not exceed 900 mg daily

(300 mg three times daily). Weight losses consisting of 12-17 pounds in 3 months are consistent with use. 5-HTP may be used until ideal weight loss is achieved.

4. Meal-replacement formulas should only be used when one cannot get to some good whole food for lunch or dinner, not both. When using meal-replacement formulas, the following guidelines will help keep the diet complete:

    ❋ The product should contain high-quality protein from grains, legumes, whey or hydrolyzed lactalbumin. Avoid casein-based formulas because casein is difficult to digest.

    ❋ The formula should contain at least a 5 gram combination of soluble and insoluble dietary fiber per serving.

    ❋ Balanced high-quality nutrition with enhanced levels of nutrients critical to weight-loss, such as chromium picolinate.

    ❋ Formula should have a low total fat content and should supply some essential fatty acids (EFAs).

    ❋ The product should contain no sweeteners, artificial flavors or other artificial food additives.[2]

Conclusion:
Celebrate the Joy of Womanhood

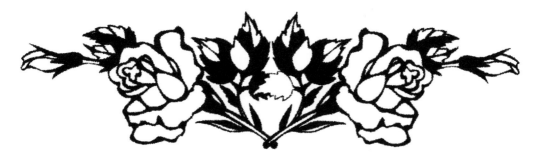

The stages of a woman's life are full of variety and great wonder. We are truly "fearfully and wonderfully made." As we move through each stage of our lives, childhood, puberty, young womanhood, menopause and finally, being "of a certain age," we can rejoice in the majesty of our Creator, be glad in the provision of bountiful, nutritious foods, and celebrate the absolute joy of being a woman. As women of God, we need not be concerned with being lesser than or equal to or superior. We may simply enjoy the honored calling in which He has placed us.

We worship Him in mind, body and spirit. Don't let your learning stop with this book; this is only the beginning. Seek to know further the intricacies of how your body functions daily, and how it changes function when you are ill. Care for your body daily by eating well, exercising, and purifying your thoughts and actions. Feed your spirit with regular communion with Christ at His table in your local church, and through the daily reading of His Word. Worship your Creator and God fervently in these ways and you will discover the truth of full health: salvation in the Lord.

"Listen to me, O house of Jacob, And all the remnant of the house of Israel, Who have been upheld by Me from birth, Who have been carried from the womb: Even to your old age, I am He, and even to gray hairs, I will carry you! I have made, and I will bear; Even I will carry, and will deliver you." *Isaiah 46: 3-4*

Resources for
Food and Products

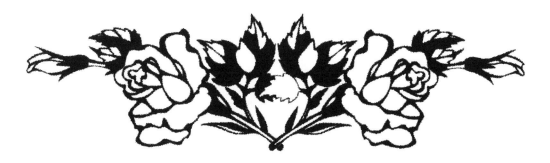

BUYING CLUB WAREHOUSES (CO-OPs)

AZURE STANDARD
79709 Dufer Valley Rd.
Dufer, OR 97021
541-467-2230
FAX: 541-467-2210
www.azurefarm.com
Organic products. Truck delivery to: OR, WA, N. ID, MT, ND
Also will ship UPS

BASIC BULK HEALTH FOODS
2617 Lackawanna St
Adelphi MD 20783
901-845-5374 phone/FAX
Organic products. Truck delivery to: NY, PA, NJ, MD, VA, WV, NC, TN, AR, AL, GA
Also will ship UPS
Contact Mike Arthur

BLOOMING PRAIRIE NATURAL FOODS
510 Kasota Ave SE
Minneapolis, MN 55414
800-322-8324 (in MN)
800-328-8241 (outside MN)
FAX: 612-378-9188
www.bpcoop.com
Organic products. Truck delivery to: MN, W. MI, E. ND, SD, WI
Also will ship UPS

BLOOMING PRAIRIE WAREHOUSE
2340 Heinz Rd
Iowa City, IA 52240
800-323-2131
319-337-6448
FAX: 319-337-4592
www.bpcoop.com
Organic products. Truck delivery to: IA, IL, IN, KS, MN, W.MI, E. ND,
NE, SD, WI, WY, OH
Also will ship UPS

COUNTRY LIFE NATURAL FOODS
PO Box 489
Pullman MI 49450
800-456-7694
616-236-5011
FAX: 616-236-8357
www.clnf.org
Organic products. Truck delivery to: MI, WI, E. MN, NE IL.
Also will ship UPS

FEDERATION OF OHIO RIVER COOPERATIVES (FORC)
320 Outerbelt St,
Columbus, OH 43213
614-861-2446
FAX: 614-861-7638
Toll-free order line for Members only.
Organic products. Truck delivery to: IN, KY, MD, NC, OH, PA, SC, TN, VA, WV

FRONTIER COOPERATIVE HERBS
3021 78th St
PO Box 299
Norway, IA 52318
1-800-669-3275
www.frontierherb.com
Organic products. National wholesale suppliers for coop and retail
Ships UPS

GENESEE FOODS
2905 Gold Rd.
Genesee, PA 16923
800-445-0094
814-228-3200
FAX: 814-228-3638
www.gnfi.com
Organic products. Truck delivery to: DE, MD, NJ, NY, OH, PA
Will also ship UPS

MOUNTAIN PEOPLES NORTHWEST
22 30th St NE Suite 102
Auburn, WA 98002
800-462-0211 (in WA)
800-336-8872 (outside WA)
FAX: 253-333-5295
Organic products. Truck delivery: AK, N. ID, MT, W. WY, OR, WA

MOUNTAIN PEOPLES WAREHOUSE
12745 Earhart Avenue
Auburn, CA 95602
800-679-6733 / 800-679-8735
FAX: 530-889-9544
Organic products. Truck delivery: CA, ID, NV, OR, UT, HI

NISHEMENY VALLEY NATURAL FOODS
Ginco Industrial Park
5 Louise Dr.
Ivyland, PA 18974
800-950-1009
215-443-5545
FAX: 215-443-7087
Organic products. Truck delivery to: CT, DE, DC, NJ, NY, PA, VA
Will also ship UPS

NORTH FARM COOPERATIVE
204 Regas Road
Madison, WI 53714
800-236-5880 fax 608-241-0688
www.northfarm.com
Organic products. Truck delivery to all of: WI, MI, IL, MN, IN
and parts of: MO, IA, OH, KY, WY, SD, ND, MT

OZARK CO-OPERATIVE WAREHOUSE
1601 Pump Station Rd.
PO Box 1528
Fayettville, AR 72702
501-521-4920
FAX: 501-521-9100
Organic products. Truck delivery to:
AL, AR, FL, GA, KS, LA, MS, OK, NC, SC, TX

SOMETHING BETTER NATURAL FOODS
22201 Capital Ave NE
Battle Creek, Michigan 49017
616-965-1199
FAX: 616-965-8500
www.somethingbetternaturalfoods.com
Also a distributor of Country Life Natural Foods
Organic Products. Truck delivery to: IN, KY, TN, NC, AL, GA, OH, IL
Will also ship UPS

TUCSON COOPERATIVE WAREHOUSE
350 South Toole Ave
Tucson AZ 85701
800-350-2667
602-884-9951
FAX: 602-792-3258
Organic products. Truck delivery to: AZ, S. CA, CO, NM, NV, W. TX, UT

WALTON FEED
135 North 10th (PO Box 307)
Montpelier, Idaho 83254
800-847-0465 or 208-847-0465
FAX: 208-847-0467
www.waltonfeed.com
Ship by truck anywhere in the US, will ship UPS

WHEAT MONTANA
PO Box 647
Three Forks, MT 59752
800-535-2798
www.wheatmontana.com
Growers and distributors of grains. Growers of Prairie Gold and Bronze Chief wheat. Ship by truck anywhere in US with minimum, will ship UPS.

Excerpted from *Naturally Healthy Living: Real Food For Real Families* © 2001 by Vickilynn Haycraft and Shonda Parker

For other cooperatives, you may send a self-addressed stamped envelope to Co-op Directory Services, ATTN: Kris Olsen, 919 21st Ave. S, Minneapolis, MN 55404. No phone calls, please. They have a free packet of information that you will find most useful, sayeth Vickilynn.

ORGANIC PRODUCE SUPPLIERS

Finding organic produce suppliers is a little more difficult than finding whole foods cooperative warehouses. Some cooperative warehouses offer organic produce as well as bulk foods and supplements. State agricultural agencies are usually good resources for finding organic farmers within one's state. One option may be contacting your local health food store and asking if your co-op could order organic produce through them at a reduced cost for volume sales. While this may not be welcomed, it doesn't hurt to ask.

COMMUNITY ALLIANCE WITH FAMILY FARMERS
PO Box 363
Davis, CA 95617
916-756-8518 or 800-852-3832 for ordering, www.caff.org
Publishes a directory, *The National Organic Directory*, selling for $44.95 + shipping & handling. This directory lists farms, wholesalers, farm suppliers, resource groups, organic standards per state, support businesses and a commodities sold and bought index per state. 386 pp.

NATIONAL INSTITUTE FOR SCIENCE, LAW AND PUBLIC POLICY
Publishes *Healthy Harvest III, A Directory of Sustainable Agriculture Organizations* that lists organic growing associations, food distributors, journals of organic farming, seed sales, training programs and so forth in the U.S. and abroad. May be purchased for $10.95 (plus $1 postage) from
Potomac Valley Press
1424 16th St., NW, #105
Washington, D.C. 20036

MAIL-ORDER HEALTHY LIVING SUPPLIERS

There are several different mail-order businesses that supply tools, supplements, kitchen equipment, whole grains, etc. The following list is by no means comprehensive. These are just the suppliers that I personally know or have purchased from in the past few years. Just because a business is listed here does not imply a Naturally Healthy™ endorsement. Educated consumers must decide for themselves whom they can support with their dollars.

The Healthy Baby Supply Company
Department D
323 W Morton Dr
St Paul MN 55107
612-225-8535
Company supplies cloth diapers, herbs for mom and baby, organic baby food, healthcare books and products.

Herbs from God's Garden
103 New Braintree Rd W
Brookfield MA 01581
508-867-6214
Organically grown and wild-crafted herbs.

Joyful Living Distributors
1601 Kelly Rd
Aledo, TX 76086
817-441-7074 or e-mail bellfamily@characternet.com
Kristy Bell and husband, Bill, have a large selection of kitchen equipment, long-storage grains, books, and food and nutritional supplement supplies.

TriLight Herbs
11358 Tyler Ft Rd
Nevada City CA 95959
800-HERB-KID or 888-HERB-MOM
www.trilightherbs.com
Mary Bennett and husband, Lyle, produce liquid herbal TincTract™s that are sold direct to moms at wholesale cost when they order in sufficient bulk quantities ($25 minimum order) to encourage mothers to stock their herbal medicine cabinet.

Self-Care Catalog
104 Challenger Dr
Portland TN 37148-1716
800-345-3371 or e-mail SlfCare@aol.com
A catalog with a large number of home health tools.

In His Hands
Home Birth Supplies
105 Lost Pine
Elgin, TX 78621
1-800-247-4045
www.InHisHands.com

Spirit-Led Childbirth
PO Box 1225
Oakhurst, CA 93644
209-683-2678 or 888-683-2678
Leslie Parrish provides a good selection of birth and parenting supplies as well as natural healthcare books and supplements.

Urban Homemaker
PO Box 440967
Aurora, CO 80044
1-800-55-BREAD or 303-750-7230 for inquiries
www.urbanhomemaker.com
Marilyn Moll and husband, Duane, have a full catalog of products, including the Liquid Light™ herbal TincTracts™ , that assist families in healthy living. Marilyn also publishes a magazine called *The Homemaker's Forum*.

NUTRITIONAL SUPPLEMENT COMPANIES

The companies listed sell primarily to health food stores or professional providers. Some sell directly to consumers. These are noted with a bold asterisk (*****).

American Health
Pearl River, NY 10965
(800) 445-7137

Maker of Super Papaya digestive enzymes as well as other products.
15 Dexter Plaza

bio/chem Research
865 Parallel Dr.
Lakeport, CA 95453
(800) 225-4345

Producers of Citricidal, a grapefruit seed extract antimicrobial.

Biotec Foods
2639 S. King St. #206
Honolulu, HI 96826
(800) 331-5888

High-potency, enteric-coated antioxidant enzyme formulas to include superoxide dismutase and glutathione peroxidase.

Blessed Herbs
109 Barre Plains Rd.
Oakham, MA 01068
(800) 489-HERB

Company providing herb tinctures, bulk herbs, oils, salves, tea bags, soaps, shampoos and books.

Cardiovascular Research/
Ecological Formulas
106 "B" Shary Circle
Concord, CA 94518
(800) 888-4585
510-827-2636 (in CA)

Advanced nutritional medicine line specializing in immune support, yeast problems and allergies.

Eclectic Institute, Inc.
11231 S.E. Market St.
Portland, OR 97216
(800) 332-HERB

Maker of Opti-Natal prenatal vitamins as well as other multiple vitamin and mineral formulas specifically designed for certain health conditions. Only source I know of that carries the freeze-dried herbal products such as nettles that have received so much research attention in the past few years.

*The Pure Body Institute
423 East Ojai Ave. #107
Ojai, CA 92303
(800) 952-PURE

Makers of the best internal cleansing program I've tried. It is gentle yet very effective. "Nature's Pure Body Program" is my personal choice for pre-pregnancy detoxification.

Enzymatic Therapy
825 Challenger Dr.
Green Bay, WI 54311
(800) 648-8211

Top-quality line of nutritional products. Michael Murray, N.D. is on their Scientific Advisory Board, which tells me this company is committed to excellence. ET has been the first to provide U.S. consumers with nutritional supplements common on the European market because of their research-proven benefits.

*Frontier Cooperative Herbs
PO Box 299
Norway, IA 52318

Full-line of bulk herbs. Now expanding their encapsulated product line.

Kal Healthway Vitamins
PO Box 4023
Woodland Hills, CA 91365
(818) 340-3035

Nutritional product company that has been around for a long time. Many times available through food co-ops.

McZand Herbal, Inc.
PO Box 5312
Santa Monica, CA 90405
(310) 822-0500

A limited line of herb supplements primarily designed for immune and respiratory support.

Metagenics, Inc./Ethical Nutrients
971 Calle Negocio
San Clemente, CA 92672
(800) 692-9400

Quality and excellence are found in this company's products that are sold under the brand of Metagenics for practitioners, Ethical Nutrients for health food stores. I especially like their line of Intestinal Care products. They have the only milk thistle extract tablets standardized to contain 80% silymarin that I have been able to find.

Miracle Exclusives, Inc.
PO Box 349
Locust Valley, NY 11560
(800) 645-6360

Floradix liquid vitamin and herb supplements are made by this company including Floradix Liquid Iron mentioned in the section on anemia.

*Mother's Choice™
11358 Tyler Foote Rd
Nevada City, CA 95959
1-888-HERB-MOM, toll-free

Excellent liquid line of herbal TincTracts™ sold directly to mothers at wholesale cost. Sister line of the Liquid Light™ herbs. Carries my midwife formulas.

Natren
3105 Willow Lane
Westlake Village, CA 91361
(800) 992-3323
(800) 992-9292 (CA)

Maker of probiotics such as "Life Start" containing *Bifidobacterium infantis* and "Bio Nate," an improved strain of *acidophilus*.

Nature's Apothecary
997 Dixon Road
Boulder, CO 80302
(303) 581-0288

Source of herbal products.

Nature's Sunshine Products, Inc.
PO Box 1000
Spanish Fork, UT 84660

A line of products sold through distributors in a multi-level organization.

Nature's Herbs
PO Box 335
Orem, UT 84059
(800) HERBALS

Owned by Twinlab, a company producing excellent herbal products certified both for potency and organic.

Nature's Way
10 Mountain Spring Pkwy.
Springville, UT 84663
(800) 9-NATURE

Superior quality nutritional and herbal products easily found in the health food store and in many food co-ops.

NF Formulas, Inc.
805 S.E. Sherman
Portland, OR 97214
(800) 547-4891

A full line of naturopathic products including my favorite prenatal supplement, Prenatal Forte. Their Echinacea products are some of the best. Professional only.

Phyto-Pharmica
   (see Enzymatic Therapy)

Progressive Labs/ ***Kordial Products**
1701 W. Walnut Hill Lane
Irving, TX
(800) 527-9512

Extensive line of dietary supplements certain to please both health practitioners and consumers due to their commitment to excellence in product and customer service.

Rainbow Light Nutritional Systems
207 McPherson St.
Santa Cruz, CA 95060

Maker of a quality line of supplements to include one of my favorite menstrual cycle (800) 635-1233 regulators, Fem-a-Gen.

Schiff Products
180 Moonachie Ave.
Moonachie, NJ 07074
(800) 526-6251

Full line of products available in many health food stores.

Standard Process Laboratories
12209 Locksley Lane, Ste. 15
Auburn, CA 95603
(800) 662-9134
(916) 888-1974 (in CA)

Extensive line of naturopathic formulas sold only to chiropractors and naturopaths. Some midwives may be able to distribute them.

Traditional Medicinals
4515 Ross Road
Sebastopol, CA 95472

A quality line of herbal teas sold for specific health conditions such as "Pregnancy Tea" and "Mother's Milk."

Tri-Light, brand name Liquid Light™
11358 Tyler Foote Road
Nevada City, CA 95959
(800) HERB-KID

My personal favorite for liquid
herbs. This company uses a
unique multi-staged process that
captures the optimum benefits from
the herbs while preserving enzymes
and preventing oxidation. Children
love the flavor (glycerine is naturally
sweet) and adults like the potency. No
alcohol, no sugar, in squeeze bottles -
standard glycerites, these are not.
Yes, they do process my Midwife Formulas,
and no, I do not receive any
financial gain from their sales. Lyle
and Mary are kind, generous Believers
concerned with family health.

Twin Labs
2120 Smithtown Ave.
Ronkonkoma, NY 11779
(800) 645-5626

A complete line of nutritional
supplements commonly found in
health food stores and food co-ops.

UAS Laboratories
9201 Penn Ave. S., #10
Minneapolis, MN 55431
(800) 422-DDS-1

Maker of the DDS Acidophilus, a
high-potency strain.

Magazines and Journals:

Herbalgram
American Botanical Council
PO Box 201660
Austin, TX 78720
(512) 331-8868
Subscriptions: $25/yr.

Herb Research Foundation
10007 Pearl St., Ste. 200
Boulder, CO 80302
*Membership to HRF is $35/yr and
includes a subscription to
Herbalgram.

Published quarterly by the
American Botanical Council
and the HerbResearch Foundation.
This is THE best source for up-to-date
research news, legal and regulatory
information regarding nutritional
supplements and the ABC mail-order
bookstore offerings include basic herbals as
well as more scientific works for
the professional herbalists (or
consumers desiring to truly
educate themselves for family herbal care).
No home considering botanical medicine
should be without this journal.

Both ABC and HRF are non-profit educational organizations and need our support to continue their very valuable work.

HRF members also receive the *Herb Research News* quarterly edited by Rob McCaleb, HRF President.

**For a small increased member donation, the Herb Research Foundation will also include a subscription to *Herbs For Health*, my very favorite herb magazine!

Quarterly Newsletter of The American Herb Association
PO Box 1673
Nevada City, CA 95959
Subscriptions: $20/yr. Quarterly.

This 20-page newsletter is always
packed with an array of information
from case studies and research news to
book reviews - my personal favorite
section. AHA is an association of
medical herbalists; however, because of
AHA's commitment to promoting
the use, understanding and acceptance
of herbs, anyone interested in herbs
will benefit from regular reading of the
Newsletter.

Digest of Alternative Medicine
PO Box 2049
Sequim, WA 98382
(360) 385-0699 (FAX)

An offshoot of the *Townsend Letter for Doctors* that is designed for use by patients. Write for subscription information.

Townsend Letter for Doctors
Townsend Letter Group
911 Tyler Street
Port Townsend, WA 98368
(360) 385-6021

This 150+ page journal is written for and by health care providers. Published 10 times per year at $49 subscription price, it is an incredible value to those interested in the technical, scientific side of nutritional healing. Many naturopathic researchers publish their findings in this journal.

BOOKS: BOTANICAL MEDICINE

The ABC Herbal by Steven Horne. Wendell Whitman Co., 302 E. Winona Avenue, Warsaw, IN 46580. 1992. 82 pp. $7.95.

A quick afternoon read that will give parents the very basics of herbal care with an obvious leaning to Thomsonian practice. The aspect I like best about this book is the guidelines for using the Tri-Light Liquid Light TincTracts (the formulas mentioned in the book are those that Tri-Light processes).

A-Z Guide to Drug-Herb-Vitamin Interactions, edited by Schuyler W. Lininger, Jr. D.C.

This book is invaluable in the home health library. The book lists common medications, how they interact with natural supplements as well as listing the natural supplements and their safety isues. A must have!

The Alternative Health & Medicine Encyclopedia by James E. Marti.

The *Encyclopedia* is basically a guide to alternative therapies. The botanical and nutritional medicine information is good; however, there are therapies I personally have a caution about using.

Antibiotic Alternative by Cindy L. A. Jones, Healing Arts Press.

How to protect yourself and your family from the misuse of antibiotics; learn how to control and overcome infections with natural remedies; and how to maintain a healthy and vibrant immune system without antibiotic dependency.

Botanical Influences on Illness: A Sourcebook of Clinical Research by Melvin R. Werbach, M.D. and Michael T. Murray, N.D., Third Line Press, Tarzana, CA. 1994. 344 pp. $39.95

This book is not a guide as to what to use or how to use it; rather, it is more an annotated bibliography that most herbalists will find most helpful when called upon to cite scientific safety and efficacy documentation for clients.

The Complete Botanical Prescriber by John A. Sherman, N.D.

A wonderful book for those who counsel others in use of herbs or for those consumers who wish to be highly informed. The price is a little steep at $59.95, but well worth it for professionals.

Dr. Murray's Total Body Tune-Up by Michael T. Murray, N.D., Bantam Books

A book to help you slow down the aging process, keep your system running smoothly and help your body's natural healing processes – for Life!

Encyclopedia of Natural Medicine by Michael Murray, N.D. and Joseph Pizzorno, N.D.

Dr. Murray and Dr. Pizzorno, authors of *The Textbook of Naturopathic Medicine* which is the definitive text for naturopathic physicians, have written this book as a comprehensive guide for consumers detailing how to use herbs, vitamins, minerals as well as diet and other nutritional supplements. The book employs an easy-to-use style which lists health conditions followed by natural treatments for said conditions.

Foundations of Health: The Liver & Digestive Herbal by Christopher Hobbs. Botanica Press, P.O. Box 742, Capitola CA. 1992. 321 pp. $12.95

Most of us might skip this book thinking *we* do not have a problem with our livers. How much we would miss if we did. The longer I practice herbal health care with an emphasis on pregnancy and childbirth, I find the liver to be an organ not to be ignored if one seeks a healthy pregnancy. Mr. Hobbs does an excellent job of explaining liver and digestive function, and his recommendations for keeping our liver happy and healthy are superb.

The Green Pharmacy by James Duke, Ph.D.

This book is a treasure chest full of wisdom in using herbs medicinally. Dr. Duke is one of the leading experts in using plants for medicine. This book combines his down-home style with specific guidelines as to which herbs are best used to treat specific illnesses. I've enjoyed this book greatly!

Gynecology and Naturopathic Medicine, A Treatment Manual by Tori Hudson, N.D.

An excellent "treatment manual" is what I would call this spiral-bound book. All practitioners who combine botanical medicine with women's health care will want this one in their library. Consumers who want to participate more in their preventive health plan than simply doing what someone else recommends without knowing why will also benefit from the reading of this book.

The Healing Herbs by Michael Castleman.

This book is a wonderful introduction to the "scientific" side of herbal medicine. Castleman lists the historical usage of herbs, herbal healing information based on scientific research, safety concerns for specific herbs where appropriate as well as herb-growing guidelines. The only thing I do not agree with in this book is the advice to not give herbal medicines to children under 2 years of age or older people over 65 or pregnant women. My own family has chosen to inform ourselves of the risks versus benefit of both herbal medicine and modern pharmaceuticals and choose herbal medicine (wise and prudent use) the majority of the time.

The Healing Power of Herbs by Michael T. Murray, N.D.

The subtitle of this book is "The Enlightened Person's Guide To The Wonders Of Medicinal Plants." Dr. Murray does not mean mystically enlightened; rather, this title appropriately refers to the scientific enlightenment that occurs when we begin to dip into the great body of research regarding botanical medicines. After reading this book, which is so well documented, one will *know* botanical medicine yields results that not only compete with modern pharmaceuticals, but actually outperform them in many instances.

Herbs for Health and Healing by Kathi Keville, Director of the American Herb Association.

Easy to read. Plenty of make your own formulas. Kathi is an authority in the professional herbalist field, and it shows in her book.

Herbal Prescriptions for Better Health by Donald J. Brown, N.D.

Currently one of my favorite herbals. Excellent scientific documentation along with well-researched toxicity information. A very readable writing style makes this book one of the most essential for families who are practicing herbal medicine at home.

Herbal Tonic Therapies by Daniel B. Mowrey, Ph.D.

Another great book due to the abundance of scientific citations for each herb discussed. The format follows herbal support for the body systems which does include a section on gynecological health which I have found particularly helpful.

Herbs of Choice by Varro Tyler, Ph.D., ScD.

Although Dr. Tyler and I would not agree on every point of what defines herbalism, I feel this book will serve as a bridge between the informed natural health community and the all-too-often misinformed medical community. This is not a "starter" book into herbal healing unless one has a command of pharmaceutical terms and a good knowledge of biochemistry. Dr. Tyler does present meticulous documentation that makes further study a breeze.

Herbs That Heal by Michael A. Weiner, Ph.D. and Janet Weiner.

This book is extremely user-friendly. A number of herbs are presented complete with their history, recent scientific findings, preparation instructions and some caution information. Since the material is not foot- or end-noted, further study proves difficult for those of us who want to see the source.

Natural Alternatives to Over-the-Counter and Prescription Drugs by Michael T. Murray, N.D.

This book is my favorite book to recommend to those who are new to botanical medicine. Dr. Murray provides excellent information about drugs commonly used for the health complaints he addresses in the book, and then he follows this with excellent lifestyle/dietary and nutritional supplement recommendations. Must have this book when practicing herbal medicine.

Natural Prescriptions by Robert M. Giller, M.D. and Kathy Matthews.

I found this book to be more about vitamins, minerals and other nutritional supplements than about botanical medicine; however, I have included it in this section because I liked the background information given on each health condition. Health problems are listed alphabetically with treatment options in a shaded box at the end of each section.

The Natural Pharmacy by Skye Lininger, D.C., Editor-in-Chief, Jonathan Wright, M.D., Steve Austin, N.D., Donald Brown, N.D., Alan Gaby, M.D.

An excellent sourcebook for specific illness recommendations, detailed information, including toxicity risk, of nutritional supplements.

Preventing Osteoporosis with Ipriflavone by Andrea Girman, M.D., M.P.H. & Carol Poole

This book helps you to discover a safe, proven alternative to estrogen replacement therapy.

BOOKS: NUTRITION

Fertility, Cycles and Nutrition by Marilyn M. Shannon. The Couple to Couple League Int'l. Cincinnati, OH. 1992. 167 pp. $10.95.

Marilyn Shannon offers in this book the basics of nutrition coupled with specific nutritional recommendations to positively affect fertility. I especially like the tone of this book — favorable to large families, breastfeeding and natural family planning.

Food - Your Miracle Medicine by Jean Carper. HarperCollins Publishers, Inc., 10 E. 53rd St., New York, NY. 1993. 528 pp.

This is my favorite and most-often reached for book on nutritional healing. The format listing disorders by body system and then alphabetically within that system is so easy to use. Even critics of "alternative medicine" cannot argue with research proving Grandma's chicken soup really is good for respiratory bugs.

Encyclopedia of Nutritional Supplements by Michael T. Murray, N.D.

Murray completely covers all nutritional supplements with information on how to obtain through diet and supplementation, correct dosages and toxicity information.

The Healing Power of Foods by Michael T. Murray, N.D. Prima Publishing, P.O. Box 1260BK, Rocklin, CA. 1993. 438 pp.

Yes, I do have every one of this man's books, and the reason is I have found every single one of them to be a source of solid education on nutrition and herbs. This particular book educates one on the nutrient content of different foods as well as provides an ample section on health conditions that may be treated with food recommendations given.

The Word on Health by Dr. Michael Jacobson, Moody Press.

This book gives a good foundation for health by looking at what we are required to do in God's Word for our health as well as our areas of freedom. One of the best books on this subject I've seen.

What Every Pregnant Woman Should Know by Gail Sforza Brewer with Tom Brewer, M.D. Penguin Books, 375 Hudson St., New York, NY. 1985. 260 pp.

The information contained in this book arms women with the nutritional guidelines that help to prevent the pregnancy complication, metabolic toxemia, of late pregnancy. While I do believe protein is important to prevent MTLP, I believe that it is beneficial to obtain said protein from a variety of sources that excludes liver.

What the Bible Says About Healthy Living by Rex Russell, M.D.

I am so thankful for this book. Finally, a book on the biblical aspects of healthy living that gives guidelines for ideal eating without placing legalistic burdens upon us in our eating practices. Consequences of poor body stewardship are discussed according to medical findings to support biblical principles without placing our body's salvation upon our eating practices. A must have for the home library!

BOOKS: PREGNANCY AND CHILDBIRTH

A Good Birth, A Safe Birth by Diana Korte & Roberta Scaer.

This is a must read for a thorough understanding of the risks and benefits regarding the technology of birth especially for those planning a hospital birth. Those planning a home birth will also benefit from this information. Do not assume having a midwife will mean no intervention; be informed.

The Birth Book. William Sears, M.D. and Martha Sears, R.N.

This is a comforting and reassuring book about the natural-ness of childbirth. The Sears clearly and simply share with us the benefits of "low-tech, high-touch" birth. Options are discussed openly and honestly. Illustrations are some of the best I've seen of birth positions. My favorite quote from the book, "While you can't totally orchestrate the perfect birth—birth is full of surprises—you can create the conditions that increase your chances of having the birth you want."

Childbirth Without Fear. Grantly Dick-Read.

Helen Wessel Nickel has revised this edition of Mr. Dick-Read's classic on natural childbirth. An excellent book for the parent-to-be.

Emergency Childbirth. Gregory White.

A small, basic manual for those who are concerned about not making it to the hospital or their midwife not making it to the home for delivery. Step-by-step instructions are clear and easy to understand.

Heart and Hands. Elizabeth Davis.

A guide written for midwives, but useful for mothers planning home-birth, on caring for pregnant women.

The Joy of Natural Childbirth, A Revised Edition of Natural Childbirth and the Christian Family. Helen Wessel-Nickel.

Helen walks one through the beginning of pregnancy to the completion of a joy-filled birth in this book. An essential book to understand God's design for birth. Keep in mind that while His design is perfect, our fallen world may yield a not-quite-perfect birth. I suppose what I am trying to say is that although pain in childbirth may not be a curse from God, most women do experience some (or a great deal of) pain during their childbirth experience. The perception of pain in daily life has an impact on the perception of pain during birth.

Under the Apple Tree. Helen Wessel Nickel.

Once again, Helen imparts to us her expansive knowledge of Christian parenting and birth. Her personal style of writing makes the book a very easy read.

Birth After Cesarean. Bruce Flamm, M.D.

Extensive documentation of the safety of vaginal birth following a cesarean section. Debunks the myth of "Once a cesarean, always a cesarean."

Understanding Diagnostic Tests in the Childbearing Year. Anne Frye.

This new revised edition is Frye's best yet. While I do not practice midwifery, therefore I am not the book's target group, I do prefer to have my own information available at home to go over my lab results and aid in self-diagnosis where possible. I found this book to be the one most referred to during my childbearing year (my midwife kept calling *me* for the answers—she didn't own the book until I sold her one of her own).

Breastfeeding

Bestfeeding. Renfrew, Fisher and Arms.

A basic guide to breastfeeding. Accurate information and helpful pictures.

Breastfeeding and Natural Child Spacing. Sheila Kippley.

Discusses and details the "ecological" method of natural child spacing. The information is accurate and scientific on the natural amenorrhea imparted through breastfeeding which I believe is God's perfect design for a woman's healing and rest for baby's first year.

Keys to Breastfeeding. William and Martha Sears.

Practical advice for new and expectant moms on nutrition, dietary needs and advantages of breastfeeding.

The Womanly Art of Breastfeeding. La Leche League International.

Don't throw out the baby with the bath water. While I may disagree with much of the childrearing information promoted through La Leche League, this organization should be recognized for being highly instrumental in a resurgence in breastfeeding in this country. Their breastfeeding support is invaluable for many women. I was told to call La Leche League when I had my first child prematurely. I did not. I now wish I had as he was bottle-fed, developed allergies and chronic ear infections until I finally got him off of formula and cow's milk.

Marriage and Family

Reforming Marriage by Douglas Wilson.

This is a wonderful book on marriage. I've never seen a clearer presentation of the Christ-Bride/Husband-Wife relationship.

The Fruit of Her Hands by Nancy Wilson.

This is an excellent book for women on "our part" in the marriage relationship.

Other family titles by Douglas Wilson: *Her Hand in Marriage, Standing on the Promises.*

BOOKS: FAMILY PLANNING

All the Way Home by Mary Pride

The Art of Natural Family Planning. John and Sheila Kippley.

The Bible and Birth Control. Charles D. Provan.

A Full Quiver: Family Planning and the Lordship of Christ. Rick and Jan Hess.

Letting God Plan Your Family. Samuel A. Owen, Jr.

Children: Blessing or Burden (Exploding Myth of the Small Family). Max Heine.

Grand Illusions: The Legacy of Planned Parenthood. George Grant.

The Way Home by Mary Pride

Notes

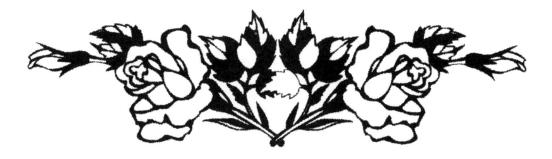

Part One, Chapter 1

[1] Kitzinger, Sheila. *The Complete Book of Pregnancy and Childbirth*, Alfred A. Knopf, NY, NY: 1990. p. 56

Part Two, Chapter 1

[1] Wilson, J. Robert and Elsie Reid Carrington. *Obstetrics and Gynecology*. The C.V. Mosby Co. St. Louis: MO, 1987. P. 49.
[2] Ibid. p. 40.
[3] Kitzinger, Sheila. *The Complete Book of Pregnancy and Childbirth*. Alfred A. Knopf. NY:NY, 1990. P. 56.

Part Two, Chapter 2

[1] Fox J et al.: The effect of hysterectomy on the risk of an abnormal screening Papanicolaou test result. Am J Obstet Gynecol. 1999; 180:1104-9
[2] Associated Press, 2000.

Part 3, Chapter 1

[1] Freudenheim, J. et al. 1994. "Exposure to breast milk in infancy and the risk of breast cancer." *Epidemiology* 5: 324-33
[2] Newcomb, P.A., et al. 1994 "Lactation and a reduced risk of pre-menopausal breast cancer." *New England Journal of Medicine* 330 (2): 81-87.

Part 3, Chapter 2

[1] Weiner, Herbs That Heal. pp. 113-114.
[2] Ibid, p. 151.
[3] Ibid, p. 276.
[4] Ibid, p. 339.
[5] Castleman, Michael. The Healing Herbs. Emmaus, PA: Rodale Press, 1991. p. 77.
[6] F. Umeda, et al., "Effect of Vitamin E on Function of Pituitary-gonadal Axis in Male Rats and Human Subjects," Endocrinol Jpn, 29(3), June 1982, p. 287-292.
[7] Crawford, Amanda McQuade. Herbal Remedies for Women. Rocklin, CA: Prima Publishing, 1997. p. 136.
[8] C.Y. Hong, et al., "Astragalus Membranaceus Stimulates Human Sperm Motility in Vitro," Am Jnl of Chin Med, 20(3-4), 1992, p. 289-294.
[9] Calloway, D. H. "Nutrition in reproductive function of man," Nutrition Abstracts and Reviews, Reviews in Clinical Nutrition, 53:5 (1983), 361-82.
[10] Piesse, J. "Zinc and human male infertility," International Clinical Nutrition Reviews, 3:2 (1983), 4-6.
[11] Jungling, M.D. and Bunge, R.G. "The treatment of spermatogenic arrest with arginine," Fert. Ster. 27 (1976), 282.

[12] Davies, Nutritional Medicine, p. 318.

[13] E. Kessopoulou, et al., "A Double-blind Randomized Placebo Cross-over Controlled Trial Using the Antioxidant Vitamin E to Treat Reactive Oxygen Species Associated Male Infertility," Fertil Steril, 64(4), October 1995, p. 825-831.

[14] S. Palmero, et al., "The Effect of L-acetylcarnitine on Some Reproductive Functions in the Oligoasthenospermic Rat," Horm Retab Res (1990 Dec) 22(12):622-6.

[15] A. Lenzi, et al., "Glutathione Therapy for Male Infertility," Arch Androl, 29(1), July-August 1992, p. 65-68.

Part 3, Chapter 3

[1] Wilson, J. Robert & Carrington, Elsie Reid. *Obstetrics & Gynecology*. St. Louis: MO: The C.V. Mosby Co., 1987. p. 210.

[2] Mowrey, Daniel B., Ph.D. *Herbal Tonic Therapies*. New Canaan, CT: Keats Publishing, Inc., 1993. pp. 312-14.

[3] Weiner, Michael A., Ph.D., & Janet A. *Herbs That Heal. Mill Valley, CA: Quantum Books, 1994. p. 135.*

[4] Castleman, Michael. *The Healing Herbs*. Emmaus, PA: Rodale Publishing, 1991. pp. 79-81.

[5] Castleman, p. 295.

[6] Weiner, p. 51.

[7] Weiner, p. 339.

[8] Kurzepa, S. & Samojlik, E. Studies on the effects of extracts from plants of the family rosaceae on gonadotropin and thyrotropin in the rat. *EndoKrinol Pol.* 14:143, 1963.

[9] Phone conversation with DeAnn Domnick. Ms. Domnick was unable to recall the naturopathic school from which the students came; therefore, I have been unable to trace the origin of the students' remark.

[10] R.S. Shah, et al., "Vitamin E Status of the Newborn in Relation to Gestational Age, Birth Weight and Maternal Vitamin E Status." *British Journal of Nutrition*, 58(2), September 1987, pp. 191-198.

Part 4, Chapter 1

[1] Null, Gary, Ph.D. *The Clinician's Handbook of Natural Healing* NY, NY: Kensington Publishing Corp. 1997. P.693.

[2] Bassett I.B., Pannowitz D. L. and Barnetson RSC, "A comparative study of tea tree oil versus benzoyl peroxide in the treatment of acne," *Med J Australia* 153: 455 - 458, '90.

[3] Lininger, Skye, Wright, Jonathan, Austin, Steve, Brown, Donald, Gaby, Alan. *The Natural Pharmacy*. Rocklin, CA: Prima Publishing, 1998. p. 6.

[4] L.H. Leung, "Pantothenic Acid Deficiency as the Pathogenesis of Acne Vulgaris," *Med Hypoth,* 44(6) June 1995, p. 490-492.

[5] M.G. Longhi, et. Al., "Activity of Crataegus Oxyacantha Derivatives in Functional Dermocosmesis," *Fitoterapia*, L(2), 1984, P. 87-99.

Part 4, Chapter 2

[1] Frye, Anne. *Understanding Diagnostic Tests in the Childbearing Year.* New Haven, CT: Labrys Press, 1993.
[2] Frye, p. 132-133.
[3] el-Chobaki, F.A., Saleh, Z.A., & Saleh, N. The effect of some beverage extracts on intestinal iron absorption. *Journal of Nutritional Sciences*, 29(4): 264-269, 1990.
[4] Null, Gary, Ph.D. *A Clinician's Handbook for Natural Healing*, p. 831.

Part 4, Chapter 3

[1] Weiner, Michael A., Ph.D. & Janet A. *Herbs That Heal.* Mill Valley, CA: Quantum Books, 1994. p. 138.
[2] Mowrey, Daniel B., Ph.D. *Herbal Tonic Therapies.* New Canaan, CT: Keats Publishing, Inc., 1993. p. 334.
[3] Tyler, Ph.D., ScD., Varro E. *Herbs of Choice.* Binghamton, NY: Pharmaceutical Products Press, 1994. p. 137.
[4] Weiner, p. 240.
[5] A.D. Genazzani, et al., "Acetyl-l-carnitine as Possible Drug in the Treatment of Hypothalamic Amenorrhea." *Acta Obstet Gynecol Scand*, 70(6), 1991, pp.487-492
[6] Wilson, J. Robert, and Carrington, Elsie Reid. Obstetrics and Gynecology. St. Louis, MO: The C.V. Mosby Company, 1987. p.115
[7] D.M. Lithgow and W.M. Politzer, "Vitamin A in the Treatment of Menorrhagia." *South African Med Jrnl*, 51(7), February 12, 1977. pp. 191-193.

Part 4 Chapter 4

[1] Murray, Michael T., N.D. *Natural Alternatives to Over-the-Counter & Prescription Drugs.* NY,NY: William Morrow & Co., 1994.
[2] Ibid.
[3] Ibid.
[4] Ibid.
[5] Weiner, Michael A. Ph.D. & Janet A. *Herbs That Heal.* Mill Valley, CA: Quantum Books, 1994. p. 154-55.
[6] Carper, Jean. *Food - Your Miracle Medicine.* NY,NY: HarperCollins Publishers, Inc., 1993. p. 311
[7] Carper, p. 314.
[8] Carper, p. 321.
[9] Castleman, Michael. *The Healing Herbs.* Emmaus, PA: Rodale Pres, 1991. p. 188.
[10] Carper, *Food - Your Miracle Medicine*, p. 322.

Part 4, Chapter 5

Source: 1995 Gaia Symposium Proceedings Book, Michael T. Murray, N.D.'s article on Anxiety and Depression.

Part 4, Chapter 6

[1] Shannon, Marilyn. *Fertility Cycles and Nutrition*. Cincinnati, OH: Couple to Couple League Int'l, Inc., 1992. p. 47-48.

Part 5, Chapter 2

[1] Crawford, Amanda McQuade. *Herbal Remedies for Women*. Prima Publishing. Rocklin:CA 1997. P. 90.
[2] Ibid.

Part 5, Chapter 3

[1] Passariello, N., Fici, F., Guigliano, D. et al. "Effects of pyridoxine alpha-ketoglutarate on blood glucose and lactate in type I and II diabetics." Internat J Clin Pharmacol Ther Toxicol 1983; 21: 252-56.
[2] Abdel-Aziz, M.T., Abdou, M.S., Soliman, D. et al. "Effect of carnitine on blood lipd pattern in diabetic patients." Nutr Rep Internat 1984; 29: 1071-79.
[3] Sotaniemi, E. A., Haapakoski, E., Rautio, A. "Ginseng therapy in non-insulin-dependent diabetic patients." Diabetes Care 1995; 18:1373-75.
[4] Yongchaiyudha, S., Rungpitarangsi, V., Bunyapraphatsara, N., Chokeshaijaroenporn, O. "Anti-diabeteic activity of Aloe vera juice. Clinical trial in new cases of diabetes mellitus." Phytomed 1996; 3: 241-43.
[5] Leatherdale, B.A., Panesar, R.K., Singh, G. et al. "Improvement of glucose tolerance due to Momordica charantia (karela)." BMJ 1981; 282:1823-24.
[6] Srivastava, Y., Venkata-krishna-bhatt, H., Verma, Y., et al. "Antidiabetic and adaptogenic properties of Momordica charantia extract: An experimental and clinical evaluation." Phytother Res 1993; 7: 285-89.
[7] Welihinda, J., Karunanaya, E, Sheriff, M.H.B, Jayasinghe, K. "Effect of Momordica charantia on the glucose tolerance in maturity onset diabetes." J Ethnopharm 1986; 17:277-82.

Part 5, Chapter 4

[1] Melnikow, J. "Natural history of cervical squamous intraepithelial lesions: A meta-analysis." Obstetrics & Gynecology 1998, 92:727-35

[2] Konno R, Paez C, Sato S, Yajima A, Fukao A HPV, histologic grade and age. Risk factors for the progression of cervical intraepithelial neoplasia. J Reprod Med 1998 Jul;43(7):561-6

[3] Rome RM, Chanen W, Pagano R *The natural history of human papillomavirus (HPV) atypia of the cervix.* Aust N Z J Obstet Gynaecol 1987 Nov;27(4):287-90

Part 5, Chapter 6

[1] *Women's Health Letter.* August 1994, p. 8.

[2] Giller, Robert M., M.D. and Matthews, Kathy. *Natural Prescriptions.* NY,NY: Carol Southern Books, 1994, p. 140.

[3] Murray, Michael T., N.D. *The Healing Power of Herbs.* Rocklin, CA: Prima Publishing, 1992, p. 207.

Part 6, Chapter 1

[1] Giller, Robert, M., M.D. & Matthews, Kathy. *Natural Prescriptions.* NY,NY: Carol Southern Books, 1994. p. 101-103.

[2] Weiner, Michael A., Ph.D. & Janet A. *Herbs That Heal.* Mill Valley, CA: Quantum Books, 1994. p. 136.

[3] Weiner, p. 79, 188, 264-265, 331-332.

[4] Sun, D.X., Abraham, S.N, Beachey, E, H "Influence of berberine sulfate on synthesis and expression of pap fimbrial adhesin in uropathogenic Escherichia coli. *Antimicro Agents Chemother* 1988; 32: 1274-77.

Part 6, Chapter 2

[1] Frye, Anne. *Understanding Lab Work in the Childbearing Year.* New Haven, CT: Labrys Press, 1991. p.381

[2] Belaiche, P. Treatment of vaginal yeast infections of *Candida albicans* with the essential oil of *Melaleuca alternifolia. Phytotherapie* 15:15-16, 1985.

[3] Brown, Donald J. *Herbal Prescriptions for Better Health.* Rocklin, CA: Prima Publishing, 1996. p.210

[4] Frye, p. 384.

[5] Mowrey, Daniel B. *Herbal Tonic Therapies.* New Canaan, CT: Keats Publishing, Inc. 1993. p. 80.

[6] M.S. Litschgi, et al., [Effectiveness of a Lacctobacillus Vaccine on Trichomonas Infection in Women. Preliminary Results], *Fortschr Med,* 98(41), November 6, 1980, p. 1624-1627.

[7] J. Starzyk, et al., " Biological Properties and Clinical Application of Propolis. II. Stidus on the Antiprotozoan Activity of Ethanol Extract of Propolis," *Arzneimittelforschung, 27(6), 1977, p. 1198-1199.*

Part 6, Chapter 3

[1] Shonda Parker as noted while working as a medical assistant for Dr. James R. Bergeron in Shreveport, LA, 1984.

2   Frye, Anne. Understanding Lab Work in the Childbearing Year. New Haven, CT: Labrys Press, 1990. p. 338.

3   Willson, J. Robert and Carrington, Elsie Reid. Obstetrics and Gynecology. St. Louis, MO: The C.V. Mosby Co., 1987. p. 609-10.

4   Varney, Helen. Nurse-Midwifery. St. Louis, MO: Blackwell Scientific Publications, Inc., 1987. p. 169.

5   Frye, Anne. Understanding Lab Work in the Childbearing Year. New Haven, CT: Labrys Press, 1990. pp. 339-40.

6   Carper, Jean. Food - Your Miracle Medicine. NY,NY: HarperCollins, Inc., 1993. p. 362.

7   Murray, Michael T., N.D.The Healing Power of Foods. Rocklin, CA: Prima Publishing, 1993. p. 307.

8   Murray, The Healing Power of Foods, p. 307.

9   Giller, Robert M., M.D. & Matthews, Kathy. Natural Prescriptions. NY,NY: Carol Southern Books, 1994. p. 184.

10 Weiner, Michael A. & Janet A. Herbs That Heal. Mill Valley, CA: Quantum Books, 1994. p. 79.

11 Weiner, p. 84.

12 Weiner, p. 97.

13 Weiner, p. 141-42.

14 Weiner, p. 276-77.

15 Weiner, p. 296.

16 Mowrey, Daniel B., Ph.D. Herbal Tonic Therapies. New Canaan, CT: Keats Publishing, Inc., 1993. p. 67, 323.

17 Weiner, p. 126, 319.

18 D.B. Mowrey, The Scientific Validation of Herbal Medicine, New Canaan, CT, Keats Publishing, 1986, p. 73.

19 M. Amoros, et al., "Comparison of the Anti-herpes Simplex Virus Activities of Propolis and 3-methyl-but-2-enyl Caffeate," Journal of Nat Prod, 57(5), May 1994, p. 644-647.

20 IuF Maichuk, et al., [The Use of Ocular Drug Films of Propolis in the Sequelae of Ophthalmic Herpes], Voen Med Zh, (12), December 1995, p. 36-39.

Part 7, Chapter 1

Sources: Dr. Whitaker's Guide to Natural Healing by Julian Whitaker, M.D. Prima Publishing: Rocklin, CA, 1995, and Herbal Prescriptions for Better Health by Donald J. Brown, N.D., Prima Publishing: Rocklin, CA, 1996.

Part 7, Chapter 2

1   Frye, Anne. *Understanding Lab Work in the Childbearing Year*. New Haven, CT: Labrys Press, 1990. p. 187.

2   Murray, Michael T., N.D. *Natural Alternatives to Over-the-Counter & Prescription Drugs*. NY,NY: William Morrow & Co., 1994. p. 101.

3   Murray, p. 102.

4   Ibid.

5   Murray, p. 113.

6   Ibid.

[7] Silagy, C., Neil, A.W. "A meta-analysis of the effect of garlic on blood pressure." *J Hypertension* 1994; 12: 463-68.

[8] Murray and Pizzorno, pp. 166-167.

[9] Murray and Pizzorno, p. 167 and 170.

[10] Fraser, G.E., Sabate, J. Beeson, W.L., and Strahan, T.M. "A possible protective effect of nut consumption on risk of coronary heart disease." *Arch Int Med* 152: 1416-24, 1992.

[11] Satyavati, G.V. Gum guggal (Commiphora mukul). "The success story of an ancient insight leading to a modern discovery." *Ind J Med Res* 87: 327-35, 1988.

[12] Nityanard, S., Srivastava, J.S., & Asthana, O.P. "Clinical trials with gugulipid, a new hypolipidaemic agent." *J Assoc Phys India* 37: 321-28. 1989.

[13] Lau, B.H., Adetumbi, M.A. & Sanchez, A. "Allium sativum (garlic) & atherosclerosis: a review." *Nutr Res* 3:119-28, 1983.

[14] Carper, Jean. *The Food Pharmacy.* NY,NY: Bantam Books, 1989.

[15] Murray, Michael T., N.D. *The Healing Power of Foods.* Rocklin, CA: Prima Publishing, 1993. p. 115-17.

[16] Arsenio, L. Bodria, P., Magnati, G., et al. "Effectiveness of long-term treatment with pantethine in patients with dyslipidemias." *Clin Ther* 8: 537-45, 1986.

[17] Gaddi, A., Descovich, G., Noseda, G. et. al. "Controlled evaluation of pantethine, a natural hypolipidemic compound, in patients with different forms of hyperlipoproteinemia." *Atheroscl* 50:73-83, 1984.

[18] Murray, Michael T., N.D. *Natural Alternatives to Over-the-Counter and Prescription Drugs.* NY, NY: William Morrow & Co., Inc., 1994. p. 140.

Part 8

[1] Murray, Michael T., N.D. *Natural Alternatives to Over-the-Counter and Prescription Drugs.* NY,NY: William Morrow & Co., 1994.

[2] ibid.

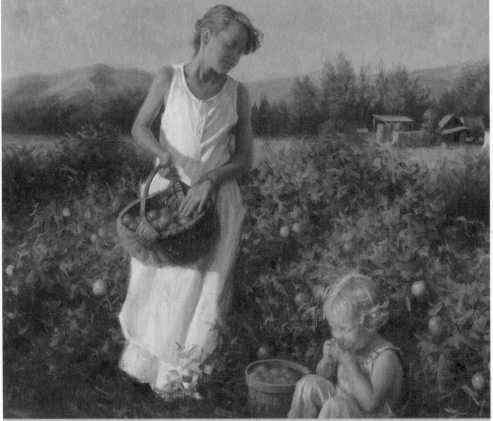

MOMMY DIAGNOSTICS™

THE NATURALLY HEALTHY FAMILY'S GUIDE TO HERBS
AND WHOLE FOODS FOR HEALTH

SHONDA PARKER

AUTHOR OF THE NATURALLY HEALTHY PREGNANCY™

FOREWORD BY DR. MARY ANN BLOCK | AUTHOR OF *No More Ritalin!*

All the information you need to safely and effectively care for your
entire family, from rocking horse to rocking chair.

$14.99 US, ISBN: 1-929125-11-9

THE NATURALLY HEALTHY PREGNANCY™

THE ESSENTIAL GUIDE TO NUTRITIONAL AND BOTANICAL MEDICINE FOR THE CHILDBEARING YEARS

SHONDA PARKER

AUTHOR OF MOMMY DIAGNOSTICS™

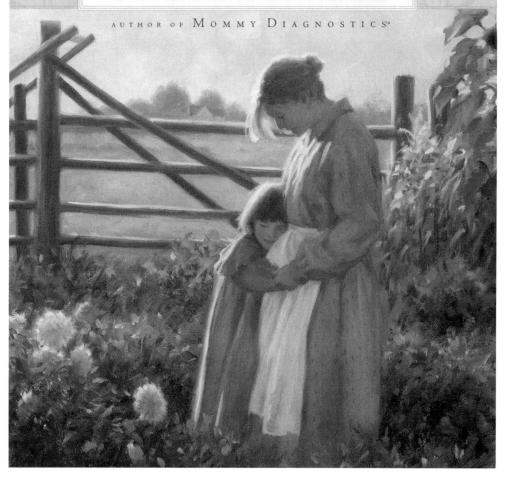

This book answers all of your questions about nutritional and herbal medicine for the childbearing years.

$14.99 US, ISBN: 1-929125-12-7